PEARLS
of WISDOM

Cardiology
BOARD REVIEW

Second Edition

Michael Zevitz, M.D.

McGraw-Hill
Medical Publishing Division

New York Chicago San Francisco Lisbon London
Madrid Mexico City Milan New Delhi
San Juan Seoul Singapore
Sydney Toronto

Cardiology Board Review, Second Edition

Copyright © 2006 by The McGraw-Hill Companies, Inc. All rights reserved. Printed in the United States of America. Except as permitted under the United States Copyright Act of 1976, no part of this publication may be reproduced or distributed in any form or by any means, or stored in a data base or retrieval system, without the prior written permission of the publisher.

3 4 5 6 7 8 9 0   CUS/CUS   0 9 8

ISBN 0-07-146422-0

> **Notice**
>
> Medicine is an ever-changing science. As new research and clinical experience broaden our knowledge, changes in treatment and drug therapy are required. The authors and the publisher of this work have checked with sources believed to be reliable in their efforts to provide information that is complete and generally in accord with the standards accepted at the time of publication. However, in view of the possibility of human error or changes in medical sciences, neither the authors nor the publisher nor any other party who has been involved in the preparation or publication of this work warrants that the information contained herein is in every respect accurate or complete, and they disclaim all responsibility for any errors or omissions or for the results obtained from use of the information contained in this work. Readers are encouraged to confirm the information contained herein with other sources. For example and in particular, readers are advised to check the product information sheet included in the package of each drug they plan to administer to be certain that the information contained in this work is accurate and that changes have not been made in the recommended dose or in the contraindications for administration. This recommendation is of particular importance in connection with new or infrequently used drugs.

The editors were Catherine A. Johnson and Marsha Loeb.
The production supervisor was Phil Galea.
The cover designer was Handel Low.
Von Hoffmann Graphics was printer and binder.

This book is printed on acid-free paper.

Cataloging-in-Publication data for this title is on file at the Library of Congress.

INTERNATIONAL EDITION ISBN: 0-07-110858-0

Copyright © 2006. Exclusive rights by The McGraw-Hill Companies, Inc. for manufacture and export. This book cannot be re-exported from the country to which it is consigned by McGraw-Hill. The International Edition is not available in North America.

DEDICATION

*To my wife Joan, the love of my life, and to my children
Erica and Laurel, who have each, in their own way,
taught me to give it my all in everything that I do.*

AUTHOR

Michael E. Zevitz, M.D.
Assistant Professor of Medicine
Finch University of Health Sciences/
The Chicago Medical School
Director, Echocardiography Lab
Iron Mountain VA Medical Center

INTRODUCTION

Congratulations! *Cardiology Board Review: Pearls of Wisdom*, Second Edition, will help you learn some Cardiology. Originally designed as a study aid to improve performance on the Cardiovascular Disease Written Boards/Recertification. This book is full of useful information. While intended for Cardiology specialists, we have learned that this unique format is also useful for Cardiology Fellows, as well as housestaff and medical students rotating through Cardiology. A few words are appropriate discussing intent, format, limitations, and use.

Since *Cardiology Board Review* is primarily intended as a study aid, the text is written in rapid-fire question/answer format. This way, readers receive immediate gratification. Moreover, misleading or confusing "foils" are not provided. This eliminates the risk of erroneously assimilating an incorrect piece of information that makes a big impression. Questions themselves often contain a "pearl" intended to reinforce the answer.

Additional "hooks" may be attached to the answer in various forms, including mnemonics, visual imagery, repetition, and humor. Additional information not requested in the question may be included in the answer. Emphasis has been placed on distilling trivia and key facts that are easily overlooked, that are quickly forgotten, and that somehow seem to be needed on board examinations.

Many questions have answers without explanations. This enhances ease of reading and rate of learning. Explanations often occur in a later question/answer. Upon reading an answer, the reader may think, "Hmm, why is that?" or, "Are you sure"? If this happens to you, go check! Truly assimilating these disparate facts into a framework of knowledge absolutely requires further reading on the surrounding concepts.

Information learned in response to seeking an answer to a particular question is retained better than information that is passively observed. Take advantage of this! Use *Cardiology Board Review* with your preferred source texts handy and open. This book does have limitations. We have found many conflicts between sources of information. We have tried to verify in several references the most accurate information. Some texts have internal discrepancies further confounding clarification.

Cardiology Board Review risks accuracy by aggressively pruning complex concepts down to the simplest kernel; the dynamic knowledge base and clinical practice of Cardiology is not like that! Furthermore, new research and practice occasionally deviates from that which likely represents the correct answer for test purposes. This text is designed to maximize your score on a test. Refer to your most current sources of information and mentors for direction for practice.

Cardiology Board Review is designed to be used, not just read. It is an *interactive* text. Use a 3 x 5 card and cover the answers; attempt all questions. A study method we recommend is oral, group study, preferably over an extended meal or pitchers. The mechanics of this method are simple and no one ever appears stupid. One person holds the book, with answers covered, and reads the question. Each person, including the reader, says "Check" when he or she has an answer in mind. After everyone has "checked" in, someone states his/her answer. If this answer is correct, on to the next one; if not, another person says their answer or the answer can be read. Usually, the person who "checks" in first gets the first shot at stating the answer. If this person is being a smarty-pants answer-hog, then others can take turns. Try it, it's almost fun! *Cardiology Board Review* is also designed to be re-used several times to allow, dare we use the word, memorization. Open round bullets are provided for any scheme of keeping track of questions answered correctly or incorrectly.

We welcome your comments, suggestions and criticism. Great effort has been made to verify these questions and answers. Some answers may not be the answer you would prefer. Most often this is attributable to variance between original sources. Please make us aware of any errors you find. We hope to make continuous improvements and would greatly appreciate any input with regard to format, organization, content, presentation, or about specific questions. We also are interested in recruiting new contributing authors and publishing new textbooks. We look forward to hearing from you! Study hard and good luck!
M.E.Z.

TABLE OF CONTENTS

PHYSICAL EXAMINATION OF THE HEART AND CIRCULATION

O   **How many phases does the jugular venous pulse have?**

Three, if the patient is in sinus rhythm.

O   **What is hepatojugular reflux and what is its significance?**

When there is right ventricular failure, sustained compression of the abdomen will cause the central venous pressure to rise. The venous neck pulses will become more prominent and their level will ascend in the neck. This is a characteristic sign of congestive heart failure, the most common cause of increased level of venous pressure in the neck veins and of exaggerated venous pulses.

O   **What is the effect of changing posture on carotid arterial pulses?**

Carotid pulses are relatively unaffected by changing posture.

O   **What is the normal ascendancy of jugular venous pulses?**

With the patient's thorax and head elevated at 45 degrees from the horizontal, the venous pulses should ascend no more than 1 or 2 cm above the level of the manubrium sterni.

O   **What is the significance of jugular venous distention?**

Jugular venous distention is a clinical measure of central venous pressure and right atrial pressure. For each centimeter of venous pulse ascension, greater than 2 cm above the manubrium sterni, this represents approximately 1 mmHg of increased pressure in the right atrium. Since the normal right atrial pressure ranges from 6-12 mmHg, a jugular venous pulse of 5 cm above the clavicle would represent a right atrial pressure of approximately 15 mmHg.

O   **What other conditions, besides congestive heart failure, does a positive hepatojugular reflux occur?**

Constrictive pericarditis, inferior vena caval obstruction, severe tricuspid regurgitation, cardiac tamponade, massive pulmonary embolus, and superior vena cava syndrome.

O   **What is the *a* wave of the venous pulse caused by?**

The "a" wave of the venous pulse is caused by atrial contraction. It is absent in atrial fibrillation, and in atrial flutter, may be replaced by rapid smaller oscillations which occur approximately 300 times per minute.

O   **What is the *c* wave of the venous pulse?**

This is still in dispute, but is felt to be the result of the bulging of the tricuspid valve at the beginning of ventricular systole. It may also be augmented by the underlying carotid arterial pulse.

○   **What is the *v* wave of the venous pulse?**

The *v* wave is a passive filling wave as blood from the periphery enters the atrium in the latter part of ventricular systole. Large V waves occur in severe mitral regurgitation, severe mitral stenosis, severe right-to-left shunts (Eisenmenger's syndrome) and in severe aortic stenosis with marked CHF.

○   **What is the x descent?**

The x descent is produced by atrial diastole.

○   **What is the y descent?**

The y descent occurs on opening of the tricuspid valve and filling of the right ventricle from the right atrium.

○   **What conditions result in a large "a" wave?**

Any condition that results in pulmonary hypertension that is transmitted back to the right ventricle and right atrium. These conditions include severe mitral regurgitation, cor pulmonale, pulmonary embolism and severe dilated cardiomyopathy. Other conditions include tricuspid stenosis, tricuspid atresia and large atrial septal defects. Certain arrhythmias can also result in large "a" waves. These include complete AV block, AV dissociation, and atrial and nodal extrasystoles. These arrhythmias produce *irregular* cannon "a" waves, as opposed to the *regular* large "a" waves of the other above-mentioned conditions.

○   **What is the significance of large c-v waves?**

It is a sign of significant tricuspid regurgitation. They may also occur in the presence of atrial fibrillation in the absence of tricuspid regurgitation.

○   **What is Kussmaul's sign and what is its significance?**

Kussmaul's sign is when there is jugular venous distention on inspiration, rather than the expected fall in venous pulse during inspiration. While it is not diagnostic of constrictive pericarditis, it occurs very commonly in constrictive pericarditis and uncommonly in pericardial tamponade, a feature that helps to clinically differentiate the two conditions. Kussmaul's sign can also occur in congestive heart failure.

○   **What other abnormality occurs in constrictive pericarditis and what other conditions can it occur in?**

A prominent y descent. A prominent x descent is also occasionally found. Again, a prominent y descent is not diagnostic of constrictive pericarditis, but it is a prominent feature in the disorder and is uncommon in cardiac tamponade.

○   **What conditions are bounding arterial pulses found?**

1.   anxiety
2.   aortic insufficiency
3.   patent ductus arteriosus, the commonest cause in children
4.   left-to-right intracardiac shunts such as sinus of Valsalva aneurysm with rupture into the right heart or coronary arteriovenous fistula
5.   thyrotoxicosis
6.   severe anemia
7.   hyperkinetic heart syndrome
8.   beriberi
9.   systemic AV fistula

10. complete AV block
11. severe peripheral vascular disease
12. hypertrophic cardiomyopathy, particularly of the obstructive type

О   **What is the significance of pulsus bisferiens?**

It is characterized by a double systolic impulse and is most prominent over the carotid artery. It is most common in combined aortic stenosis and insufficiency, but can be seen in patients with isolated aortic insufficiency and obstructive hypertrophic cardiomyopathy.

О   **What is pulsus tardus and what is its significance?**

Pulsus tardus is a delayed, slow carotid upstroke that is typically found in severe aortic stenosis.

О   **What is pulsus paradoxus and what conditions is it found in?**

Pulsus paradoxus is an exaggerated inspiratory fall in blood pressure during quiet breathing. When the inspiratory fall in systolic blood pressure exceeds 8-10 mmHg, it is abnormal. It occurs in constrictive pericarditis in a third to one-half of cases. It occurs in an overwhelming majority of cases of cardiac tamponade. It also occurs in asthma and emphysema, and rarely in cardiomyopathy.

О   **Which valve closes first in the cardiac cycle in a normal patient, the mitral valve or tricuspid valve?**

The mitral valve.

О   **What conditions cause a loud first heart sound (S1)?**

Mitral stenosis (unless very severe), short PR interval, exercise, tachycardia, anemia and hyperthyroidism.

О   **What conditions cause a faint first heart sound (S1)?**

Very severe mitral stenosis (virtually immobile valve leaflets, mitral insufficiency, 1° AV block, and severe hypertension.

О   **What conditions is there wide splitting of the second heart sound?**

Right bundle branch block, pulmonic stenosis and atrial septal defect (due to late closure of the pulmonic valve), and mitral insufficiency and ventricular septal defect (due to early closure of the aortic valve).

О   **What condition causes fixed splitting of the second heart sound?**

Atrial septal defect.

О   **What conditions cause paradoxical splitting of the second heart sound?**

Left bundle branch block, aortic stenosis, patent ductus arteriosus, obstructive hypertrophic cardiomyopathy and occasionally during myocardial ischemia.

О   **What conditions cause narrow splitting of the second heart sound?**

Right-to-left intracardiac shunt with right heart failure (Eisenmenger's complex).

О   **What is an opening snap and what is the significance of the time between the second heart sound and the opening snap?**

An opening snap is heard in 90% of patients with mitral stenosis and is a sharp, high-pitched closure sound heard best at the apex, after the second heart sound. The shorter the duration between the second heart sound and the opening snap, the more severe the mitral stenosis and the higher the left atrial pressure.

○ **What is the murmur of aortic stenosis?**

A systolic ejection, crescendo-decrescendo murmur, heard best at the apex and aortic area, radiating to the carotids and unchanged by respiration. The murmur increases in intensity with increased inotropy, increased preload and increased afterload.

○ **What is the murmur of mitral stenosis?**

A low-pitched diastolic rumble with an opening snap, best heard at the apex.

○ **What is the murmur of aortic regurgitation?**

A decrescendo, high-pitched diastolic murmur heard best at the lower left sternal border, starting almost with the second heart sound.

○ **What is the murmur of mitral regurgitation?**

A holosystolic, high-pitched murmur that starts with the first heart sound and continues through the second heart sound, best heard at the apex and radiates either to the axilla or lower left sternal border.

○ **What is the murmur of mitral valve prolapse?**

A mid-systolic high-pitched murmur best heard at the apex and left sternal border, accompanied by one or more systolic clicks in half the cases.

○ **What is a pericardial friction rub and what does it sound like?**

A pericardial friction rub is a high-pitched, scratchy, almost sandpaper-like sound with two or three components, occurring in both systole and diastole, that occurs in pericarditis, and is best heard with the patient leaning forward or lying prone in deep expiration. Pericardial friction rubs may disappear and return within minutes.

CARDIAC HEMODYNAMICS AND FUNCTION

○ **What is the significance of large pulmonary V waves on the pulmonary capillary wedge tracing?**

Abnormally large V waves, greater than 10 mmHg greater than the mean pulmonary wedge pressure, represent filling of the left atrium during systole against an abnormally large left atrial pressure. It is most commonly found in mitral regurgitation, but can also be seen in mitral stenosis, congestive left ventricular failure, ventricular septal defects, Eisenmenger's complex, and, in rare instances, severe aortic regurgitation.

○ **What is the arteriovenous difference?**

Arteriovenous difference is the extraction of oxygen from the circulation across a given organ or tissue.

○ **What is the extraction reserve?**

Extraction reserve is the factor by which the AV difference can increase at a constant blood flow.

○ **What is the arterial oxygen saturation in a normal human? Venous saturation?**

The arterial saturation in a normal human is 95%. The venous saturation in a normal human is around 75%, but differs slightly, depending on where you measure.

○ **What is the normal AV difference for oxygen in man?**

40mL per liter of blood.

○ **What is the normal extraction reserve for oxygen?**

Three. This means that, given adequate metabolic demand, the body's tissues can extract three times the AV difference for oxygen, or 120mL per liter of blood. This also means that oxygen extraction increases as cardiac output falls until AV oxygen difference has tripled and cardiac output has fallen to one-third of its normal value. Thereafter, further reduction of cardiac output will result in tissue hypoxia, anaerobic metabolism, acidosis, and eventually, circulatory collapse.

○ **What is the normal cardiac output in an adult human?**

Approximately 4-6 L/min, depending on numerous factors such as body size, metabolic rate, posture, age, body temperature, anxiety, environmental heat and humidity and a host of other factors.

○ **What is the most accepted method of expressing cardiac output?**

Cardiac index. Cardiac index is the cardiac output divided by the body surface area in square meters.

○ **What is the Fick method of determining cardiac output?**

15

Cardiac output = measured oxygen consumption/AV oxygen difference. In actual practice, the rate at which oxygen is taken up from the lungs is not measured, but rather the uptake of oxygen from room air is measured. Furthermore, the AV oxygen difference is not measured directly, but oxygen saturations of blood taken from the pulmonary artery and systemic arterial blood are sampled. The saturations are respectively converted to oxygen contents by multiplying the oxygen saturation percentage and a theoretic oxygen carrying capacity (patient's hemoglobin x 13.6). The difference in arterial oxygen content and pulmonary artery oxygen content is the AV oxygen difference.

❍ **When is the pulmonary venous blood oxygen saturation not approximated accurately by the systemic arterial oxygen saturation?**

When there is a right-to-left intracardiac shunt.

❍ **When do intracardiac shunts become physiologically important?**

When the pulmonary blood flow exceeds 1.5 to 2 times the systemic flow.

❍ **Which method of calculating cardiac output is more accurate and reliable, Fick or thermodilution method?**

Fick. Thermodilution method is easier to perform, but is prone to significant overestimation of cardiac output at low-flow, low cardiac output states.

❍ **What is the formula for estimation of systemic vascular resistance?**

SVR = (mean systemic arterial pressure – mean right atrial pressure) x 80/cardiac output.

❍ **What is the formula for estimation of pulmonary vascular resistance?**

PVR = (mean pulmonary artery pressure – mean left atrial pressure) x 80/pulmonary blood flow. Pulmonary blood flow is assumed to be equal to the cardiac output unless there is a shunt between the pulmonary and systemic circulations or an intracardiac shunt.

❍ **What is the Gorlin formula for the calculation of a stenotic aortic valve area?**

Aortic valve area (cm^2) = (cardiac output/heart rate) x systolic ejection period/44.3 x square root of mean aortic valve gradient.

❍ **What is the Gorlin formula for the calculation of a stenotic mitral valve area?**

Mitral valve area (cm^2) = (cardiac output/heart rate) x diastolic filling period/37.7 x square root of mean gradient across mitral valve.

❍ **What is the Hakki formula?**

It is a simplified valve formula that cancels out the Gorlin equation constant, systolic ejection period or diastolic filling period and the heart rate. It closely approximates the valve area calculated by the Gorlin formula.
Valve area (cm^2) = cardiac output/square root of the mean gradient.

❍ **What is the normal value for systemic vascular resistance?**

800-1400 dynes-sec-cm^{-5}.

O   A 71 year-old male is admitted with hypotension, tachypnea and tachycardia. His HR is 122, systemic blood pressure is 83/48 and the respiratory rate is 28. A Swan-Ganz pulmonary artery catheter is inserted and the cardiac output is 9.3 L/min. The pulmonary capillary wedge pressure is 11 mmHg and the SVR is 550 dynes-sec-cm^{-5}. What is this hemodynamic picture consistent with?

Distributive shock, secondary to sepsis.

O   What is the diagnosis of a patient with the following hemodynamic profile on Swan-Ganz hemodynamic monitoring: cardiac output- 3.4 L/min, PCWP- 6 mmHg, SVR- 1990 dynes-sec-cm^{-5}?

Hypovolemic shock.

O   A 71 year-old gentleman presents to the hospital with increasing shortness of breath, orthopnea, PND, and palpitations. He has a long history of recurrent CHF. His physical exam reveals bibasilar rales and he is hypotensive with a BP of 70/40 mmHg. Right heart catheterization reveals the following: cardiac output- 2.6 L/min, BSA 1.9 m^2, PCWP 34 mmHg, SVR 2100 dynes-sec-cm^{-5}, PA pressure of 65/36 mmHg, and a right atrial pressure of 37 mmHg. What is the diagnosis?

Cardiogenic shock from left heart failure.

O   In the above patient, what is the preferred drug of choice for this problem?

Dobutamine. This will reduce SVR and PCWP and potentially increase cardiac output. However, it is doubtful this patient will survive, given the profound cardiac depression found in this patient.

O   In the above patient, what is the expected pulmonary artery oxygen saturation?

40-50%. Remember, as cardiac output falls, oxygen extraction increases by the same proportion.

O   What is the most widely used hemodynamic measure of myocardial contractility?

dP/dt, the maximum rate of rise of left ventricular systolic pressure.

O   What is left ventricular stroke work?

Left ventricular stroke work is a reasonably good measure of left ventricular systolic function in the absence of left ventricular volume or pressure overload conditions, both of which may substantially increase calculated LV stroke work. Left ventricular stroke work (LVSW) may be calculated, in the absence of LV pressure tracings, by the following formula: LVSW = (mean aortic systolic pressure – mean pulmonary capillary wedge pressure) x stroke volume x .0136. This calculation is a close approximation of LV systolic function in the absence of severe mitral or aortic regurgitation. Since mean systemic arterial pressure closely approximates the mean aortic systolic pressure, one can use the following formula: LVSW = (mean systemic pressure – mean pulmonary capillary wedge pressure) x stroke volume (cardiac output/heart rate) x .0136.

O   What is the normal LVSW in adults?

90 +/- 30 gm-m.

O   What is the LVSW in patients with dilated cardiomyopathy? In patients with severe LV failure?

LVSW is often less than 40 gm-m in patients with dilated cardiomyopathy and often less than 25 gm-m in patients with severe left ventricular failure. When LVSW is less than 20 gm-m, death is expected.

O   What is the major drawback to LVSW as a measure of LV systolic function?

LVSW is a measure of <u>total</u> LV systolic function and can be considered to be a reflection of myocardial contractility only when the ventricle is reasonably homogeneous in its composition, as in most patients with dilated cardiomyopathy. In patients with marked regional wall motion abnormalities, as in coronary artery disease, particularly after myocardial infarction, LVSW may be depressed even though there remain well perfused areas of myocardium with normal contractility.

○   **What is the formula for LVSW when one has LV pressure tracing measurements?**

LVSW = (mean LV systolic pressure – mean LV diastolic pressure) x stroke volume x .0136.

○   **What is the LV stroke work index (LVSWI)?**

The LVSW, indexed to body surface area. It normally ranges from 35 gm-m/M^2 to 70 gm-m/M^2.

○   **What is the point where exercising muscle begins anaerobic metabolism?**

Anaerobic threshold (AT).

○   **At the anaerobic threshold, pulmonary CO_2 output increases with respect to O_2 consumption, reflecting CO_2 produced by buffering _____ _____.**

Lactic acid. This is also called the lactate threshold as lactate rises or the bicarbonate threshold as bicarbonate decreases.

○   **In exercise, oxygen consumption and cardiac output (CO) increase. Oxygen consumption increases more, so the (a-v) O_2 difference _____.**

Increases, due to decreased mixed venous O_2. Fit subjects achieve greater increases in both oxygen consumption and CO, and have a more reduced mixed venous O_2 at maximal exercise.

○   **Increased cardiac output in exercise is due to increased _____ _____ and _____.**

Stroke volume (SV) and heart rate. Stroke volume increases over the lower one third of the work range; further increases in cardiac output are by rate only. Cardiac output is the cardiovascular limit to exercise.

○   **What happens to $PaCO_2$ in exercise?**

Below AT, it is normal. It is reduced above AT due to the ventilatory response to lactic acidosis. In COPD, $PaCO_2$ may rise with exercise.

○   **What happens to PaO_2 in exercise?**

Usually normal, but may decrease in patients with lung disease.

○   **What is the maximal O_2 consumption?**

The O_2 consumption at which O_2 consumption plateaus despite increased power. This is the most important measure of fitness, but may be difficult to achieve. The peak O_2 consumption at maximal exercise is often used instead.

○   **What are the criteria for peak O_2 consumption?**

The patient should appear tired, or be near predicted maximal heart rate or predicted maximal minute volume. A lactate level over 8 mEq/L or RQ over 1.15 are other criteria.

○ **At anaerobic threshold, minute ventilation and CO_2 output increase with respect to O_2 consumption. The ratio of minute ventilation to O_2 consumption rises, while the ratio of minute ventilation to CO_2 output is stable, and RQ is about 1. This method of determining anaerobic threshold is the _____ _____.**

Ventilatory equivalent or ventilatory threshold.

○ **The other method of determining AT is the V-slope, comparing the CO_2 output - O_2 consumption relationship. Before AT it is linear, at AT the slope of the relation _____.**

Increases. The point at which the slope increases is the AT by the V-slope method.

○ **The difference between the maximal voluntary ventilation (measured or calculated) and the minute volume at maximal exercise is the _____ _____.**

Breathing reserve (BR). Patients with lung disease have a low BR, so at maximal exercise they are near their maximal ventilatory volume.

○ **What is the heart rate reserve?**

The heart rate reserve (HRR) is the difference between the predicted maximum heart rate and the rate at maximal exercise.

○ **O_2 delivery is reduced in heart disease, so anaerobic threshold is _____.**

Reduced. Anaerobic metabolism begins at lower workloads. Either AT or maximal O_2 consumption can be used to classify severity of heart disease.

○ **What is the normal AT (anaerobic threshold)?**

50-60% of predicted maximum O_2 consumption. Less than 40% implies circulatory impairment or deconditioning.

○ **How are heart rate and O_2 consumption related?**

Linearly. Cardiac patients may have a high rate for a given load, resulting in a left shifted heart rate - O_2 consumption relation.

○ **What does the O_2 pulse reflect?**

Stroke volume. Reduced in cardiac disease.

○ **Why is a peak O_2 consumption less than 10 ml/kg/min an indication for heart transplant?**

When due to cardiac disease, this level shows severe impairment and predicts poor survival without intervention. Levels more than 20 indicate minimal functional impairment.

○ **What are the clinical uses of cardiopulmonary exercise testing in lung disease?**

Evaluation of dyspnea and exercise limitation, assess severity, response to therapy, disability evaluation, oxygen titration.

○ **What happens to maximal work rate and oxygen consumption in COPD?**

Decreases. This pattern is common to COPD, ILD, cardiac disease, and the unfit.

O   **What is the relation between work rate and oxygen consumption in COPD?**

Normal, so the oxygen cost of work is normal, unlike the deconditioned, in which it is increased.

O   **What happens to maximum heart rate in COPD?**

Normal or reduced. The heart rate for submaximal work is increased, but maximum rate achieved is often lower than predicted.

O   **What happens to the oxygen saturation during exercise in COPD?**

Increases, decreases, or remains unchanged.

O   **T/F: In COPD breathing reserve is reduced and heart rate reserve is usually increased.**

True. This is generally true in chronic lung disease. Cardiac patients have a normal breathing reserve and variable heart rate reserve.

O   **T/F: Anaerobic threshold less than 40% in COPD suggests concomitant cardiovascular disease.**

True.

O   **What is the best test of impairment in disability testing?**

Peak or maximal O_2 consumption. Anaerobic threshold my also be used. If maximal consumption is less than 15 ml/kg/min, the patient is unable to do most jobs. 15 to 25 correlates with moderate work. Over 25, the patient can do most jobs.

O   **What is the target heart rate?**

Normally about 60% of the maximal heart rate designed by incremental exercise testing and limited by symptoms.

O   **What are the negative effects of PEEP on cardiovascular function?**

PEEP may reduce cardiac output by reducing venous return, by increasing pulmonary vascular resistance, and by shifting the interventricular septum to the left, thus reducing the left ventricular end diastolic volume.

O   **What are three ways that "best" PEEP can be determined?**

Compliance, oxygenation, and cardiac output.

O   **What is the role of corticosteriods in ARDS?**

Several studies have failed to show any benefit for the use of steroids in ARDS. There is some evidence that there may be a danger in using steroids in ARDS associated with sepsis. There is some evidence to suggest that in certain cases, in the late phases of ARDS steroids may reduce the fibrosis associated with late ARDS.

O   **What interventions have been shown to reduce the mortality of ARDS?**

Although a great number of studies have been done to reduce the mortality of ARDS, to date the only strong evidence for reduced mortality is in the computerized protocol for management of ventilator support.

Other studies on a variety of interventions in the inflammatory cascade including prostaglandins and steroids have failed to show benefit. There is recent interest in the use of prone positioning for patients with ARDS.

O   **What are the most common presenting findings in ARDS?**

Tachypnea and hypoxemia.

O   **What are the NIH criteria for the diagnosis of ARDS?**

PaO_2/FiO_2 ratio < 200, bilateral infiltrates, wedge pressure < 18.

O   **What is the cause of hypoxemia in ARDS?**

Increase in alveolar fluid causing reduced diffusion of oxygen into capillaries. thus increasing the shunt.

O   **What is the mortality of ARDS?**

Most series show a mortality of 40-60%. Some research protocols have shown a reduction to 25-30%.

O   **What are the most risk factors for ARDS?**

Sepsis, trauma, aspiration, multiple transfusions, shock, pulmonary contusions. However, many other systemic and local insults may trigger ARDS.

O   **Why is the pulmonary artery wedge pressure an important feature in the diagnosis of ARDS?**

The presence of a significantly elevated wedge pressure implies that the pulmonary edema may be hydrostatic and therefore due to left ventricular dysfunction rather than alveolar or pulmonary dysfunction and ARDS— that is, noncardiogenic pulmonary edema.

O   **Does PEEP improve ARDS?**

PEEP commonly improves oxygenation; however, it does not reduce the amount of total lung water, which is the marker for the amount of pulmonary edema present.

O   **What is the distribution of pulmonary edema in ARDS?**

Routine chest x-ray appears to show a diffuse distribution. However, CAT scan studies reveal an increased involvement in the dependent portions of the lung fields.

O   **What are the x-ray findings in ARDS?**

Diffuse ground-glass-like infiltrates that do not follow anatomical boundaries, usually bilateral.

O   **What complications are associated with ARDS?**

Barotrauma leading to pneumothorax, pulmonary infection, pulmonary hypertension, multisystem organ failure.

O   **What are the three phases of ARDS?**

Acute or exudative (up to 6 days), proliferative phase (4 to 10 days), chronic or fibrotic phase (after 7 days).

O   **What are the cellular mediators involved in the development of ARDS?**

Macrophages-TNF, monocytes-il1, endothelial cells-arachidonic acid.

○   **What is the role of PEEP in ARDS?**

Maintain alveolar inflation and functional residual capacity.

○   **What is the most feared complication associated with Extra Corporeal Membrane Oxygenation?**

Intracranial hemorrhage.

○   **Decompensated shock is characterized by what two features?**

Hypotension and low cardiac output.

○   **Oxygen delivery (DO2) can be calculated using what formula?**

Arterial oxygen content x cardiac output x 10.

○   **Arterial oxygen content (ml O2/dl blood) is calculated by using what formula?**

Hemoglobin concentration (g/dl) x 1.34 ml O2/gm hemoglobin x oxygen saturation.

○   **In hypovolemia from hemorrhage, the blood pressure is maintained until?**

The blood volume falls by 25% to 30%.

○   **What are the four factors that determine myocardial shortening?**

Afterload, preload, contractility, and heart rate and cardiac rhythm.

○   **How does preload affect myocardial shortening?**

The greater the preload, the stronger the contraction and the greater the extent of myocardial shortening.

○   **How does afterload affect myocardial shortening?**

The greater the afterload, the less the myocardial shortening.

○   **How does myocardial contractility affect myocardial shortening?**

At a constant preload and afterload, increased myocardial contractility results in greater extent and velocity of myocardial shortening.

○   **How does heart rate affect myocardial shortening?**

Within wide limits, with increasing rate, there is enhancement of contractility, and therefore myocardial shortening.

○   **What is the most accurate measure of left ventricular end-diastolic pressure?**

In the absence of mitral stenosis, the pulmonary capillary wedge pressure is the most efficient method of measuring LVEDP, as the PCWP accurately reflects left atrial pressure, which is equal to LVEDP. However, the most accurate measure of LVEDP is during left heart catheterization with direct pressure measurement of the LV.

◯   What is the most accurate method of measuring ventricular chamber volumes and segmental wall motion?

Left ventriculography using angiographic techniques.

◯   **How does the injection of contrast during left ventriculography affect cardiac hemodynamics, such as preload, afterload, contractility and heart rate?**

Contrast agents increase preload and heart rate within 30 seconds of the injection, and depress myocardial contractility. The effect on afterload is negligible. These changes can last for up to two hours after the injection during left ventriculography. Non-ionic contrast minimize these adverse effects, and are usually safer for patients with pre-existing marked elevations in LVEDP or depressed cardiac function.

◯   **How is ejection fraction calculated?**

Ejection fraction = stroke volume/end diastolic volume.

◯   **How is the regurgitant fraction calculated?**

Regurgitant fraction = stroke volume (total) – stroke volume forward/stroke volume (total).

Total stroke volume is determined by angiography and forward stroke volume is determined by the Fick method or indicator dilution method.

◯   **How does chronic volume overload and chronic pressure overload affect left ventricular mass?**

Chronic pressure overload, such as that in hypertension or aortic stenosis, results in an increase in left ventricular mass resulting from augmentation of wall thickness with little change in chamber volume (concentric hypertrophy). Chronic volume overload, such as that seen in aortic or mitral regurgitation, in primary myocardial disease, results in an similar increase in left ventricular mass resulting from ventricular chamber dilatation with only a slight increase in wall thickness (eccentric hypertrophy).

◯   **What is max dP/dt of the left ventricle and what is its significance in relation to contractility, preload and afterload?**

DP/dt max is the maximum rate of rise of ventricular pressure and is highly sensitive to acute changes in contractility. In the absence of severe left ventricular myocardial depression or marked arterial vasodilatation with very low arterial diastolic pressure, dP/dt max can be considered a reliable measure of contractility, provided preload is constant. However, dP/dt max is very sensitive to preload changes and this sensitivity is greater in ventricles with enhanced contractility and reduced in depressed ventricles. With preload held constant, increases in dP/dt max reflect an increase in myocardial contractility and decreases reflect a decrease in myocardial contractility.

◯   **T/F: Left ventricular systolic performance and contractility are the same?**

False. Systolic performance of the left ventricle is influenced by ventricular configuration, preload and afterload. Thus, it is possible to have abnormal systolic performance despite normal contractility when LV afterload is excessive, such as in accelerated or malignant hypertension. Alternatively, left ventricular systolic performance may be nearly normal despite decreased myocardial contractility if left ventricular afterload is low, as in mitral regurgitation or septic shock.

◯   **What is the best quantification of left ventricular systolic performance?**

Ejection fraction.

○   **What is the best quantification of left ventricular systolic function?**

Effective ejection fraction, as determined by the forward stroke volume divided by the LV end-diastolic volume. The effective ejection fraction is relatively independent of end-diastolic volume, and therefore, represents functional emptying of the ventricle.

ACUTE MYOCARDIAL INFARCTION

○ **How much myocardial damage from an acute myocardial infarction is necessary to result in congestive heart failure?**

Congestive heart failure is usually evident clinically if more than 25% of the left ventricle is infarcted.

○ **How much functional loss of left ventricular myocardium is required to result in cardiogenic shock?**

40%.

○ **What three secondary processes resulting in myocardial deterioration occur following acute myocardial infarction?**

Ventricular remodeling, typically following Q-wave infarctions; infarct expansion, occurring most frequently from anterior-apical infarctions and results in thinning of the left ventricular wall; and ventricular dilatation, an early and progressive response to acute myocardial infarction that is an important predictor of increased mortality following myocardial infarction.

○ **What factors play a role in the peak incidence of myocardial infarction being from 6 AM to noon?**

Blood pressure, coronary arterial tone, blood viscosity, circulating catecholamines and platelet aggregability increase on awakening and assumption of an erect posture.

○ **What is the most common cause of death related to acute myocardial infarction?**

Ventricular fibrillation, occurring within the first hour following symptoms.

○ **What percentage of patients with acute myocardial infarction develop cardiogenic shock?**

10%.

○ **What percentage of patients who are found to have myocardial infarction by other objective means, such as cardiac enzymes or radionuclide imaging studies, have normal initial ECG's?**

10%.

○ **What is the mortality among patients with their first myocardial infarction?**

2-3% in patients under 40 years of age, 7-10% in patients between 70-80 years of age, and 32% in patients older than 80 years of age.

○ **What percentage of arteries successfully opened with thrombolytic therapy for acute myocardial infarction, reocclude?**

15% of arteries successfully opened reocclude during the first few days following thrombolytic therapy.

O   **What is the mortality benefit from aspirin alone in acute myocardial infarction with thrombolytic therapy and in subsequent reinfarction?**
Aspirin reduced mortality from acute myocardial infarction by 23% and reduced non-fatal reinfarction by 49%. When used with thrombolytic therapy, there was a 40-50% reduction in mortality from acute myocardial infarction.

O   **A 63 year-old gentleman presents to the Emergency department with moderate substernal chest pressure and lightheadedness for 90 minutes. His BP on admission is 80/40 and his HR is 110/min and regular. Physical exam reveals JVD to the angle of the jaw, a right parasternal S3 gallop, an apical S4 gallop and clear lungs on auscultation. ECG reveals 2 mm ST elevation in leads II, III, and aVF with reciprocal ST depression in V1-V3. What is the most likely diagnosis and what is the most appropriate initial therapy?**

Inferior myocardial infarction with right ventricular infarction. Following 160-325 mg of aspirin administration, thrombolytic therapy, and a large bolus of intravenous saline followed by a moderately high infusion rate of saline are indicated. If the patient remains hypotensive despite adequate intravenous saline, as measured by the development of lung congestion on auscultation, intravenous Dobutamine is indicated.

O   **A seventy-year-old man is admitted to the hospital with chest pain of 3 hours duration. ECG demonstrates anterior ST elevation for which he is given aspirin, r-TPA, heparin and intravenous nitroglycerin. His symptoms resolve. Serum chemistries reveal a peak CPK of 1800 and a CK-MB fraction of 15%. He is eventually transferred out of the CCU and his hospitalization is uneventful until day 5, when he develops sudden, severe shortness of breath. BP is 110/75 and his pulse is 125 and regular. Examination reveals a new systolic murmur. What would the most appropriate therapeutic intervention be?**

Intravenous sodium nitroprusside. This patient is most likely suffering from rupture of the left ventricular septum and subsequent defect, a not uncommon complication of MI. Afterload reduction is key to stabilization until surgical repair of the VSD can be performed, usually in about 8-12 weeks, after the infarct has healed. If nitroprusside fails to stabilize the patient, intra-aortic balloon counterpulsation and intravenous nitroglycerin should be employed.

O   **A 60 year-old patient suffers an acute inferior myocardial infarction. Three hours after he arrives in the hospital, he develops ventricular fibrillation and is successfully defibrillated back to normal sinus rhythm within 30 seconds. He makes a full recovery and has no further post-MI complications. What does his ventricular fibrillation episode indicate with regard to his subsequent risk of sudden death?**

This episode has no bearing on his subsequent risk of sudden death. Ventricular fibrillation in the immediate setting of an acute myocardial infarction has no prognostic significance.

O   **A 65 year-old female presents to the hospital with sudden crushing chest discomfort and moderate shortness of breath. Her initial ECG reveals 2mm ST depression in leads V1-V4 with inverted T waves. She has bibasilar rales in the lower half of both lungs on auscultation. CXR reveals moderate pulmonary edema. Serial ECG's and CPK's confirm a non-Q wave myocardial infarction. With diuretics, her pulmonary edema resolves within 24 hours. What is the most appropriate management strategy at this point?**

Cardiac catheterization with coronary angiography. A non-Q wave MI that results in pulmonary edema signifies a large amount of myocardium at risk for reinfarction within the next year.

O   **What arrhythmias that occur in patients with acute myocardial infarction require temporary pacing?**

Complete heart block (3° AV block); new LBBB; new bifascicular block; marked sinus bradycardia with ischemic pain, hypotension, CHF, frequent PVC's or syncope despite atropine; and Mobitz II type 2° AV block.

○   A 54 year-old gentleman admitted two days ago with an acute anterolateral myocardial infarction suddenly develops atrial fibrillation with a ventricular rate of 135/min. He subsequently complains of substernal chest discomfort. His BP is 135/70. What is the most appropriate immediate action to be taken?

Synchronized DC cardioversion.

○   What percentage of patients with acute myocardial infarction develop paroxysmal atrial fibrillation?

10-15%.

○   T/F: The presence of occasional PVC's is a reliable predictor of ventricular fibrillation following acute myocardial infarction.

False.

○   A 58 year-old gentleman is admitted with an acute anteroseptal myocardial infarction. He is in pulmonary edema clinically, confirmed by CXR. His blood pressure is 122/76, his HR is 122. Despite two doses of 80 mg of intravenous furosemide, he remains in pulmonary edema. A Swan-Ganz pulmonary artery catheter is inserted and his initial hemodynamics reveal a cardiac output of 3.1 L/min and a pulmonary capillary wedge pressure of 27 mmHg. What is the most appropriate pharmacologic agent in this setting?

Intravenous Dobutamine, at a dose of 5 to 20 mcg/kg/min.

○   What is the mortality of cardiogenic shock in acute myocardial infarction?

>70%.

○   What is the incidence of rupture of the free wall of the left ventricle in patients with acute myocardial infarction?

10%. It is almost always fatal, occurring between 1 and 5 days following infarction.

○   What percentage of patients with acute myocardial infarction develop left ventricular aneurysms?

10%. 80% of LV aneurysms are located in the anterior-apical segment and result from occlusion of the left anterior descending artery.

○   What percentage of patients with acute anterior-apical Q wave infarctions develop LV mural thrombi?

50%. Over half develop mural thrombi within the first 24 hours.

○   What percentage of patients with acute myocardial infarction have a clinically evident embolic event?

4%, most within the first week following infarction.

O   **What is the current recommended therapy for patients with large anterior myocardial infarctions?**

Reperfusion therapy with thrombolytics, beta-blockers, intravenous nitroglycerin, and ACE inhibitors to limit and retard ventricular remodeling. Intravenous heparin in a sufficient dose to prolong the APTT to 1.5 to 2.0 times control should be started on admission and continued to discharge. In patients with large akinetic apical segments or mural thrombi, oral anticoagulation with warfarin is indicated for 3-6 months.

O   **What is the significance of pericarditis following acute myocardial infarction?**

Pericarditis occurs in about 20% of patients with acute myocardial infarction, more likely in Q-wave infarcts than non-Q wave infarcts. Patients with pericarditis usually have significantly larger infarcts, lower ejection fractions, and a higher incidence of congestive heart failure. The presence of pericarditis and/or pericardial effusion following acute myocardial infarction is associated with a higher mortality.

O   **A previously healthy 65 year-old man is admitted with an acute inferior myocardial infarction. Within several hours, he is hypotensive (BP 90/60), and oliguric. Insertion of a pulmonary artery catheter reveals the following pressures: pulmonary artery wedge pressure, 3 mmHg; pulmonary artery, 21/3 mmHg; and mean right atrial pressure, 11 mmHg. What is the best treatment for this man?**

Fluids, until his wedge pressure is between 16-20 mm Hg.

O   **What is the most common biologic process that causes acute myocardial infarction?**

Atherosclerotic plaque disruption, consisting of a combination of plaque ulceration, fissuring and rupture, followed by hemorrhage into the plaque, followed by the formation of a thrombus at the site of rupture. The thrombus continues to enlarge and propagate, leading to a sudden, prolonged, total occlusion of the coronary and cessation of blood flow to the supplied myocardium, resulting in myocardial necrosis if coronary occlusion lasts greater than 30 minutes.

O   **What is the earliest functional abnormality following acute myocardial infarction?**

Impaired diastolic function resulting in decreased left ventricular compliance.

O   **What compensatory contractile mechanisms occur following acute myocardial infarction in order to maintain normal cardiac output?**

Hyperkinesis of non-infarcted myocardial segments, resulting from increased circulating catecholamines and increased diastolic loading. These compensatory effects usually subside within 2 weeks, and there may be some recovery of wall motion of the infarcted segment, particularly if there was early reperfusion.

O   **Infarct expansion occurs most commonly in what type of myocardial infarctions?**

Antero-apical infarction, resulting in thinning of the left ventricular wall. It is associated with a higher incidence of complications such as congestive heart failure, cardiac rupture and left ventricular aneurysm.

O   **What physiologic changes that are affected by circadian variation play a role in an increased incidence of myocardial infarction from 6 A.M. to noon?**

Increased blood pressure, increased coronary arterial tone, increased circulating catecholamines and increased platelet aggregability.

O   **What two groups of patients are more likely to present with "silent" myocardial infarction?**

Patients with diabetes mellitus and the elderly.

O   **Moderate to heavy physical exertion and emotional stress or excitement are temporally related to the onset of symptoms in what percentage of patients with acute myocardial infarction?**

About 50%.

O   **What is the median time between onset of symptoms and arrival at a hospital in patients with acute myocardial infarction?**

Two to five hours.

O   **What is the most useful test for the immediate confirmation of the diagnosis of acute myocardial infarction?**

The electrocardiogram. It is diagnostic of acute myocardial infarction in about two-thirds of patients.

O   **What percentage of patients with confirmed acute myocardial infarction, determined by other objective means, have a normal initial ECG?**

10%.

O   **What is the normal sequential changes in the electrocardiogram during the first several days following a Q wave myocardial infarction?**

1) "Hyperacute," symmetrical, peaked T waves, 2) ST-segment elevation, 3) loss of R wave amplitude in the infarct-related leads, 4) development of Q waves in the infarct-related leads, 5) return of the ST-segment to baseline, and 6) progressive inversion of the T wave.

O   **What is the usual time sequence of the onset, peak and duration of the elevation of CK-MB levels in an acute myocardial infarction?**

CK-MB levels are usually elevated within 4-6 hours following the onset of acute myocardial infarction, peak at approximately 18-24 hours and usually return to normal at 36-48 hours following an uncomplicated infarction.

O   **At what time frame do LDH levels peak following acute myocardial infarction?**

24-48 hours.

O   **What isoforms or subforms of CK-MB have been identified, and how are they useful in detecting acute myocardial infarction?**

CK-MB activity is equally divided between a plasma form (MB-1) and a tissue form (MB-2). An increase in the normal 1 to 1 ratio of MB-2 to MB-1 to >1.5 has been shown to correlate highly with acute myocardial infarction. It is also useful in differentiating myocardial necrosis from insignificant elevation of total CK-MB in the presence of a normal total CK. An increase in the ratio of CK-MM3 (tissue form) to CK-MM1 and CK-MM2 (plasma forms) is also useful in the early and reliable diagnosis of acute myocardial infarction. Other biochemical methods of early detection of acute myocardial infarction include myoglobin and cardiac troponin T.

O   **What is the most reliable and useful method of evaluating the extent of an acute myocardial infarction?**

Two-dimensional echocardiography.

O   **What is the most important strategy for treating patients with acute myocardial infarction?**

Early reperfusion with either intravenous thrombolytic therapy or immediate primary percutaneous transluminal coronary angioplasty (PTCA).

O   **How much myocardial necrosis in an acute Q wave myocardial infarction is completed within 1 hour after the onset of symptoms? Within 2 hours? Within 4 hours?**

50%, 75% and 95% percent, respectively.

O   **What are the absolute contraindications to intravenous thrombolytic therapy?**

Major surgery, organ biopsy or major trauma within 2 weeks; significant GI or GU bleeding within 2 months; known or suspected aortic dissection; known or suspected pericarditis; known intracranial tumor; previous neurosurgery or hemorrhagic cerebrovascular accident at any time; acute severe hypertension (>200 mm Hg systolic or >120 mm Hg diastolic; head trauma within one month; thrombotic cerebrovascular accident within two months; and active internal bleeding, excluding menses.

O   **What are the relative contraindications to intravenous thrombolytic therapy?**

Mild to moderate hypertension (>180 mm Hg systolic and/or >110 mm Hg diastolic); cardiopulmonary resuscitation for < 10 minutes; puncture of non-compressible vessel; recent TIA's; thrombotic cerebrovascular accident between 2 to 6 months ago; diabetic retinopathy; active peptic ulcer; known bleeding diathesis or current anticoagulant usage; pregnancy; and exposure to streptokinase or APSAC within the last 6-9 months (does not apply to prospective t-PA administration).

O   **Which age group has the greatest reduction in mortality following the administration of thrombolytic therapy in the presence of an acute myocardial infarction?**

Patients over the age of 65, and more specifically, those patients over age 75.

O   **Previously, there had been concerns over increased likelihood of intracranial hemorrhage following the administration of thrombolytic therapy in patients over age 75. What are the respective incidences of intracranial hemorrhage following the administration of thrombolytic therapy in patients under age 75 and over age 75?**

The overall incidence of intracranial hemorrhage in patients under age 75 is 1%, slightly higher with t-PA, as opposed to streptokinase or APSAC. The overall incidence of intracranial hemorrhage in patients over age 75 is 1.3%, again slightly higher with t-PA, as opposed to streptokinase or APSAC.

O   **What are the two most common and serious side effects of streptokinase and APSAC?**

Hypotension and hypersensitivity reaction, which is antigen mediated and manifested by vomiting, itching, and swelling.

O   **What is the rethrombosis rate following the administration of t-PA without the concomitant use of intravenous heparin?**

20-30%.

O   **What is the rethrombosis rate following the administration of streptokinase in the absence of intravenous heparin administration following the completion of streptokinase therapy?**

15-20%.

O   **What is the rethrombosis rate following the administration of APSAC in the absence of subsequent intravenous heparin use?**

10%.

O **What is the rationale for intravenous heparin administration being started concomitantly with t-PA administration?**

Because the plasma clearance time of t-PA is 4-8 minutes, the coronary rethrombosis rate in the absence of intravenous heparin is significantly increased and ranges between 20-30%. With concomitant heparin administration and continued heparinization for at least 24 hours following t-PA therapy, the coronary rethrombosis rate is reduced to approximately 5-10%.

O **What is the 90-minute infarct-related coronary artery patency rate following the administration of "front-loaded" or accelerated intravenous t-PA in acute myocardial infarction, assuming concomitant administration of intravenous heparin and oral aspirin?**

80-90%.

O **What is the 90-minute infarct-related coronary artery patency rate following the administration of intravenous streptokinase in acute myocardial infarction, assuming concomitant aspirin administration?**

55-70%.

O **What is the 90-minute infarct-related coronary artery patency rate following the administration of intravenous APSAC in acute myocardial infarction, assuming concomitant aspirin administration?**

70-80%.

O **In the GUSTO-1 trial, what was the percentage of grade TIMI-3 (normal) flow occurring in infarct-related arteries following the administration of accelerated t-PA with intravenous heparin, compared to streptokinase and intravenous heparin?**

TIMI-3 flow was present at 90 minutes in 54% of infarct-related arteries with accelerated t-PA, compared to 32% of infarct-related arteries in the streptokinase group.

O **T/F: The frequency of hemorrhagic stroke following the administration of t-PA was statistically similar to the frequency of hemorrhagic stroke following the administration of streptokinase in patients under age 70.**

True.

O **T/F: The frequency of hemorrhagic stroke following the administration of t-PA was statistically similar to the frequency of hemorrhagic stroke following the administration of streptokinase in patients over age 75.**

False. The incidence of hemorrhagic stroke following the administration of t-PA was statistically higher than that following the administration of streptokinase. The overall incidence of hemorrhagic stroke in patients over age 75 receiving streptokinase is 1.1%, and 1.5% in patients over age 75 receiving t-PA.

O **Which of the thrombolytic agents, administered to patients with acute myocardial infarction, preserves left ventricular function the most?**

Except for the GUSTO-1 trial, left ventricular function, measured within the first week, as well as after one month, was similar, regardless of the thrombolytic agent used. In the GUSTO-1 trial, left ventricular function paralleled the patency rates at 90 minutes, and the group that received accelerated t-PA and intravenous heparin had slightly better left ventricular function, post-infarct, that the group that received streptokinase or the combination of streptokinase and standard dose t-PA.

O   **Which adjunctive pharmacologic therapies have been shown to improve both short-term and log-term survival following acute myocardial infarction?**

Aspirin, beta-blockers and ACE inhibitors, when given within the first 24 hours after the onset of symptoms, have all been shown to improve short-term survival following an acute myocardial infarction. Aspirin, beta-blockers and ACE inhibitors, when started between 24 hours and seven days following an acute myocardial infarction, have been shown to improve long-term survival following an acute myocardial infarction. Intravenous heparin, when administered with or immediately after thrombolytic therapy, has been shown to improve short-term survival following an acute myocardial infarction. Calcium channel blockers, nitroglycerin or nitrates, and intravenous or oral magnesium have not been shown to improve either short-term or long-term survival in acute myocardial infarction.

O   **A 57 year-old gentleman with hypertension and diabetes mellitus presents to your hospital's Emergency department with abrupt onset of crushing substernal chest pressure radiating to the jaw. His blood pressure is 75/40, his pulse is 132, his respiratory rate is 36. His lung exam reveals bibasilar rales in the lower half of both lungs, and he has both severe JVD and an S3 gallop. His electrocardiogram shows 4mm ST segment elevation in leads V1 through V6. He has never had a myocardial infarction in the past. His symptoms began 45 minutes ago. What should be the favored treatment regimen for this patient?**

If your hospital has a catheterization laboratory and it is unoccupied, this patient should undergo immediate coronary angiography with immediate PTCA of the culprit vessel. If your hospital does not have a catheterization lab, thrombolytic therapy should be immediately administered and hemodynamic support with an intra-aortic balloon counterpulsation should be strongly considered.

O   **A 63 year-old gentleman presents to your hospital with substernal chest tightness of 45 minutes duration. His electrocardiogram reveals 1.5 mm ST depression in leads I, aVL, and V4-V6. Should you give him thrombolytic therapy if he has no contraindications?**

No. Patients with non-Q wave myocardial infarctions and those with unstable angina, who eventually rule out for myocardial infarction do not appear to benefit from thrombolytic therapy. These patients should be started on intravenous heparin, given aspirin, and if they do not have pulmonary edema on initial presentation, should be started on Diltiazem.

O   **What is the acute mortality of patients with non-Q wave myocardial infarction?**

2-3%, as opposed to 10% for Q wave infarction.

O   **What percentage of patients with acute myocardial infarction will develop transient supraventricular arrhythmias?**

33%.

O   **What percentage of patients with acute myocardial infarction develop atrial fibrillation?**

10-15%.

O   **What is the preferred agent of choice in the treatment of atrial fibrillation occurring in the setting of acute myocardial infarction?**

Beta-blockers. Alternative agents, such as procainamide or amiodarone, are particularly useful in converting atrial fibrillation to sinus rhythm.

O   **A 60 year-old woman presents to your hospital with substernal chest tightness and her electrocardiogram reveals acute ST elevation in the anterior leads, consistent with an acute myocardial infarction. She is given aspirin, t-PA, beta-blockers and heparin. She is hemodynamically stable and not in heart failure. Her cardiac monitor shows 4-6 PVC's per minute with rare couplets. Should she receive lidocaine "prophylactically"?**

No. The risk-benefit ratio is unfavorable in this setting, and occasional PVC's are an unreliable predictor of ventricular fibrillation following an acute myocardial infarction. Lidocaine may also block the "escape" rhythm of accelerated idioventricular rhythm that occurs with coronary reperfusion, thus, creating a potentially life-threatening event.

O   **What is the percentage of rupture of the free wall of the left ventricle occurring in patients who die as a result of acute myocardial infarction?**

10%. This event occurs between 1 and 5 days following infarction and is almost always fatal.

O   **A 66 year-old woman has sudden onset of substernal chest pressure and comes to the Emergency Department. Her electrocardiogram and cardiac enzymes confirm an acute anterior myocardial infarction. On admission, she is hemodynamically stable, but on day 3, she develops sudden shortness of breath and she is noted to have a blood pressure of 85/50. On physical exam, she is noted to have an loud apical holosystolic murmur, bibasilar rales and an S3 gallop at the apex. A Swan-Ganz pulmonary artery catheter is placed and the pulmonary capillary wedge pressure tracing shows prominent V waves. What is the diagnosis?**

Partial or total rupture of a papillary muscle with severe mitral insufficiency.

O   **In the above patient, what is the best way to confirm the diagnosis?**

Two-dimensional and color flow Doppler echocardiography.

O   **In the above patient, what is the preferred treatment?**

Aggressive vasodilator therapy, insertion of an intra-aortic balloon counterpulsation device, and then emergent repair of the papillary muscle and mitral valve apparatus. Mortality with medical treatment alone, in this setting, is 80-90%.

O   **What is the treatment of a patient with right ventricular infarction who is hypotensive?**

Volume expansion to an optimal LV filling pressure, then cautious administration of intravenous Dobutamine.

O   **What percentage of patients with acute myocardial infarction develop left ventricular aneurysms?**

10%.

O   **Where are most left ventricular aneurysms located and what is the cause?**

80% of left ventricular aneurysms occur in the anterior-apical segment of the left ventricle. They are discrete, thin, bulging, non-contractile segments of the left ventricle that are akinetic or dyskinetic during systole. Their development is related to ventricular remodeling and they result mostly from occlusion of the left anterior descending coronary artery.

O   **What are some of the complications that may arise from the development of left ventricular aneurysms?**

Development of mural thrombi occurs in about one-half of patients with acute anterior-apical Q wave infarctions, with the resultant five-fold increase in the likelihood of embolic events. Other complications include congestive heart failure and serious ventricular arrhythmias.

○   **What percentage of patients with acute myocardial infarction have a clinically evident embolic event?**

About 4%, most often during the first week following infarction.

○   **Should anticoagulation be routinely administered to patients with acute myocardial infarction?**

For large anterior myocardial infarctions, it is currently recommended to administer intravenous heparin, until discharge, in a dose sufficient to prolong the APPT to 1.5 to 2 times normal. Those patients with a mural thrombus or a large akinetic apical segment should be treated with warfarin for three to six months. Long-term anticoagulation is generally indicated in patients with a dilated, severely hypokinetic left ventricle.

○   **Pericarditis occurs in what percentage of patients with acute myocardial infarction?**

10-20%, as defined by the presence of a friction rub.

○   **What is the significance of infarct-related pericarditis?**

Patients with infarct-related pericarditis usually have larger infarcts, have lower post-MI ejection fractions, and a higher incidence of congestive heart failure and serious ventricular arrhythmias. Patients with infarct-related pericarditis and/or the presence of pericardial effusion have a higher mortality, again related to infarct size.

○   **What is the most important prognostic determinant following acute myocardial infarction?**

Infarct size.

○   **What is the most important post-infarct diagnostic strategy following acute myocardial infarction?**

Pre-discharge non-invasive testing to risk stratify patients into those low-risk and those who are at High risk to develop non-fatal or fatal reinfarction or sudden death from arrhythmias. Many advocate pre-discharge submaximal treadmill testing, particularly in those who received thrombolytic therapy, so long as the patient did not have post-infarct angina, congestive heart failure, hypotension or serious arrythmias. Those patients with post-infarct angina, congestive heart failure, post-infarct silent ischemia as measured by ST depression, and serious arrhythmias, should undergo pre-discharge cardiac catheterization and/or further intervention (e.g., antiarrhythmic therapy, PTCA, or CABG). Some advocate symptom-limited treadmill exercise testing, instead of submaximal testing, before discharge, and there is good evidence that this is safe. Symptom-limited stress testing, either on a treadmill, or pharmacologic stress, with supplementary imaging techniques using technetium-99m sestamibi or thallium, or echocardiography, should be carried out between 10 days and 6 weeks following acute myocardial infarction in those patients deemed low-risk at discharge. Those patients with abnormal post-infarct stress tests should be referred for cardiac catheterization and, if warranted, revascularization.

○   **What percentage of patients who received thrombolytic therapy for acute myocardial infarction have single vessel disease and a total occlusion of the infarct-related artery?**

15%.

O   **What percentage of patients who received thrombolytic therapy for acute myocardial infarction have a patent infarct-related artery with a less than 50% stenosis?**

15%.

O   **What percentage of patients who received thrombolytic therapy for acute myocardial infarction have single vessel disease and > 50% stenosis in the infarct-related artery?**

35%.

O   **What percentage of patients who received thrombolytic therapy for acute myocardial infarction have a patent infarct related vessel and 2- or 3-vessel disease?**

30%.

O   **What percentage of patients with acute myocardial infarction, who receive thrombolytic therapy, have left main disease and a patent infarct-related artery?**

5%.

O   **What is the concept of "stunned myocardium"?**

This refers to muscle that is hypocontractile as a result of a brief ischemic insult but is still viable. In this situation, progressive recovery of contractile function following reperfusion may occur severa hours to weeks after the ischemic insult. This recovery occurs without revascularization from PTCA or CABG.

O   **What is the concept of "hibernating myocardium"?**

Hibernating myocardium refers to a chronically hypoperfused and hypocontractile left ventricular segment that improves functionally only after coronary revascularization.

O   **Are thrombolytic agents effective in non-Q wave MI?**

No, there is no evidence to support their use. In fact, some published data suggest that their use may be detrimental.

O   **What is the prognosis of patients presenting with Q-wave MI complicated by acute mitral regurgitation?**

Prognosis is quite compromised with an approximate one-year survival of only 50%.

O   **A 68 year-old man with a history of angina at three blocks exertion presents with onset of chest pain typical of his angina occurring after breakfast. He says this is his usual pain except that it has never occurred at rest. Physical exam is unremarkable, and the ECG reveals only non-specific findings. His pain is relieved with IV nitroglycerine and a dose of metoprolol. Laboratory findings: Total CK 110 (upper limit of normal is 150), CK-MB is 10% (upper limit of normal is 6%). What is the patients prognosis?**

The patient appears to have unstable angina and does not meet the criteria for thrombolytic therapy. However, the CK findings suggest he actually developed a non-Q wave MI. The diagnosis remains unclear in this circumstance. Whatever the diagnosis, the prognosis is <u>worse</u> in these patients compared to that of patients with unstable angina without CK-MB elevation. Thus, these patients are probably better off if evaluated as if the diagnosis is non-Q wave MI.

O   **A 77 year-old man presents complaining of chest pain. He states that he was playing racquetball, and slipped and hit his head on the wall. After this he noted the onset of chest pain**

radiating to the arm. A hot shower did not relieve his symptoms. He notes that he has continued to have a dull ache in his chest. He also reports an episode of diaphoresis after the shower and mild nausea. ECG reveals acute anterior wall MI. What would you do to treat him?

Administer aspirin immediately. The choice for additional therapy is complicated by the presence of head trauma. In the proper setting, direct PTCA is the treatment of choice, since it produces higher TIMI-3 flow rates and defines the coronary anatomy, with lower stroke risk. The benefits of direct PTCA over thrombolytic therapy, while still debated, required a high volume operator and access to a lab within 60-90 minutes. If direct PTCA was not available for this patient, the decision to give thrombolytic therapy is a difficult one.

O   **A 58 year-old woman without past medical history presents with complaints of one day of dull ache in the center of her chest that is unrelieved with aspirin or antacids. She states that the day prior to admission she had about three hours of severe discomfort in the chest associated with sweating which resolved spontaneously and she is now left with the symptoms described. Her blood pressure is 120/80, pulse is 100 and she is mildly diaphoretic. A pan-systolic murmur is heard at the left sternal border. Her lungs are clear. ECG reveals Q-Waves in leads VI-V4. Over the next twelve hours, you note that she becomes cold and clammy to palpation with signs of decreased peripheral perfusion. Her lungs remain clear. What is the diagnosis?**

Acute ventricular septal defect. Patients with acute mitral regurgitation usually have pulmonary congestion, making this diagnosis less likely. Risk factors for development of VSD include: First infarction, female gender and hypertension. Despite pathological reports that VSD most often occurs about day 4 post-myocardial infarction, clinical observations suggest that the risk is higher in the first 24 hours. Definitive treatment is surgical, but operative mortality ranges from 20 to 70%. The diagnosis should be confirmed by echocardiography. Following this, vasodilator therapy with nitroprusside and insertion of an intra-aortic balloon-pump and Swan-Ganz catheter should be performed.

O   **What affects ventricular remodeling?**

Ventricular remodeling is the change in size , shape, and thickness of both the infarcted and non-infarcted regions of myocardium. The primary factors determining remodeling are: Infarct size, scar formation, and left ventricular filling pressure. The contribution of the latter may be part of the explanation of the effect of act inhibitors in preserving left ventricular function when administered in the peri-infarct setting.

O   **What is infarct expansion?**

An increase in the size of the infarct zone unrelated to additional myocardial necrosis. Causes may include: slippage of the muscle bundles, disruption of the normal cellular array, and tissue loss in the infarct zone. This occurs almost exclusively in transmural MI's, is more common in anterior infarction, and the degree of expansion may be related to pre-existing wall thickness (hypertrophy may be protective). Infarct expansion has been shown to be associated with increased mortality and increased incidence of non-fatal complications.

O   **What are the major precipitants of AMI?**

In over half of patients with AMI, no precipitantant can be identified. However, some precipitating factors which have been identified include: emotional stress, surgical procedures, neurological disturbances and perhaps extreme physical exertion. Circadian changes in plasma catecholamines and cortisol may also play a precipitating role.

O   **What are the most common presenting symptoms of AMI?**

Chest pain. Unlike aortic dissection, this pain often waxes and wanes, and over time will become severe. It usually lasts greater than 30 minutes and is frequently described as crushing, constricting, or as pressure. The pain is typically retrosternal, and frequently radiates to the jaw and the ulnar aspect of the left arm. In some patients, particularly the elderly, AMI may present as a symptoms of acute left ventricular failure rather than chest pain.

O   **What are the other typical symptoms of AMI?**

Diaphoresis, apprehension, sense of doom, and nausea and vomiting, which occurs in greater than 50% of patients with transmural infarction. These latter symptoms, and perhaps the others to some extent, occur presumably due to the Bezold-Jarisch reflex. Nausea and vomiting occur more frequently in inferior myocardial infarction.

O   **What are the chief differential diagnoses of AMI?**

Acute pericarditis, aortic dissection and acute GI illness. Acute pulmonary embolism and costochondritis are also frequently considered in the differential.

O   **What are the most common atypical presentations of AMI?**

Congestive heart failure, angina without a prolonged or severe episode, and atypical pain location.

O   **What is a silent AMI?**

Population studies suggest that 20 to 60% of non-fatal MI's are unrecognized by the patient and are found on subsequent routine ECG. About one-half of these MI's are truly silent with no identifiable symptoms recalled by the patient. Unrecognized or silent infarction occurs more often in patients without previous anginal syndromes and is more common in diabetics and hypertensive patients.

O   **What are the most common physical findings in AMI?**

There really aren't any, and findings depend upon the absence or presence of acute complications such as congestive heart failure, acute mitral regurgitation, or cardiogenic shock. Most patients will appear to be in some distress. Of note, a fourth heart sound is almost universally present in patients with acute MI.

O   **Describe the characteristic pattern of creatine phospkokinase (CK-MB) elevation in AMI.**

CK exceeds normal levels in 4 to 8 hours after onset of MI. The mean peak for CK is 24 hours, but can range from 8 to 58 hours. Peak levels occur earlier in patients who receive reperfusion therapy, with mean peak CK rise occurring at approximately 12 hours. In general, CK levels normalize 3 to 4 days after onset of pain.

O   **What are the main causes of false positive CK elevation?**

Muscle disease, alcohol intoxication, diabetes mellitus, skeletal muscle trauma, vigorous exercise, convulsion, PE, and thoracic outlet syndrome.

O   **Describe the characteristic pattern of lactate dehydrogenase (LDH) elevation after onset of AMI?**

Levels exceed normal by 24 to 48 hours after AMI onset, peak 3 to 6 days after onset and normalize 8 to 14 days after onset. Total LDH, while sensitive, is not specific. Fractionation into its isoforms increases specificity, since myocardium contains primarily LDH-1, where other sources contain primarily the other LDH isoforms. Thus, an LDH-1 to LDH-2 ratio of greater than 1.0 is a commonly used cutoff for diagnosing recent MI. Use of LDH analysis should be limited to those patients with normal CK measurements.

O   **What other serum markers are important in diagnosing AMI?**

Recently, it has been shown that the troponins demonstrate high concordance with CK-MB, and they appear a bit earlier in the course of MI. Also, subsets of the troponins are highly specific for myocardial damage. Lastly, recent published data suggest that the amount of troponin released may be an independent marker of survival.

○ What are the most common findings on chest X-ray in AMI?

The chest X-ray is often normal, but pulmonary vascular congestion and cardiomegaly are the most common abnormalities found.

○ How sensitive is the ECG for detecting AMI?

The initial ECG is 50 to 70% sensitive for AMI. Serial ECG's increase the sensitively to about 80%. The presenting ECG is important in determining the acute treatment. All patients with suspected AMI should receive aspirin. ST-elevation AMI or new left bundle branch block are generally considered for reperfusion therapy.

○ What defines high risk EDG changes in AMI?

Anterior location, previous MI, and complex ectopy.

○ What is the differential diagnosis of "ischemia at a distance"?

ST-depression in a territory subtended by a coronary artery other than the one presumed to be responsible for the ST elevation diagnostic of MI is termed ischemia at a distance. The differential diagnosis: true ischemia, reciprocal ECG changes without ischemia, or, in the case of anterior ST depression with inferior infarction, posterior wall infarction.

Importantly, differentiation cannot be reliable made by ECG or even vectorcardiography. Surprisingly, regardless of whether the ECG changes represent ischemia in another territory or electrocardiographic changes only, they imply a worse prognosis.

○ Does the use of thrombolytic therapy in the pre-hospital setting result in better reperfusion rates?

Probably not. Although not well studies, data from several trials suggest that a thorough pre hospital assessment, including 12 lead ECG, which prepares the receiving Emergency department for the patient, saves enough time that pre-hospital thrombolysis is unnecessary. There are some trials, however, which did show some advantage to pre-hospital thrombolytic administration. In addition, where a hospital is greater than 60 minutes away, pre-hospital thrombolysis may be advantageous.

○ What factors contribute to defining patients at high risk for complications from thrombolytic therapy? (This is not the same as contraindications).

Advanced age, systolic blood pressure greater than 200 and/or diastolic blood pressure greater than 110 that is not effectively lowered with medical therapy in the emergency department, history of definite stroke, and recent surgery. There are many other factors which add incremental risk, such as CHF, hypotension, and anterior locations, to name a few. It should be noted that high risk patients receive the greatest benefits from thrombolytic therapy.

○ What are key findings of the GUSTO-I trial as related to choice of thrombolytic agent?

GUSTO-I showed that accelerated t-PA provided a 14.5% relative risk reduction in 30 day mortality compared with streptokinase. The absolute risk reduction for mortality was 1%. This was seen in patients receiving thrombolytic therapy within 4 hours on onset of chest pain. Stroke occurred slightly less frequently in streptokinase-treated patients, and the difference reached statistical significance in patients greater than 75 years of age.

○   **Routine use of oxygen is or is not beneficial in acute MI?**

The rationale is that hypoxemia is bad for myocardial necrosis and that ventilation perfusion mismatch is common in patients with acute MI, particularly after heparin administration. However, the routine use of oxygen in non-hypoxemic patients has not been proven beneficial. Regardless, most centers recommended routine use of oxygen per 6 to 12 hours to ensure adequate oxygenation of the patient.

○   **What are the major contraindications to beta-blocker therapy in AMI?**

All patients with AMI should be considered for beta-blocker therapy, and only patients with a major contra-indication should be excluded. These contraindications include: pulmonary edema with rales greater than one-third of the lung fields, marked hypotension, PR-interval greater than .24 seconds or advanced hear block, bradycardia (heart rate less than 55-60/min), or known bronchospasm (active, or history of severe bronchospasm). Several studies have repeatedly shown that beta-blocker therapy reduces mortality and recurrent ischemia when administered early in acute myocardial infarction.

○   **Which agent for the treatment of AMI has the best cost-benefit ratio with regard to improve survival?**

Aspirin. When all MI's are considered, overall acute mortality is about 13 to 14%. Administration of aspirin reduces this to about 10 to 11% (a relative reduction of about 20%). The only thrombolytic agent studied without concomitant aspirin use was streptokinase, which reduced mortality to about 10.4% The combination of aspirin plus thrombolytic agent has reduced overall mortality to 7-8 %.

○   **What are the indications for temporary transvenous pacing in AMI?**

Temporary pacing is indicated in patients at high risk with developing complete heart block, particularly new bifascicular bundle branch block or LBBB. Patients who develop a systole, Mobitz type II and complete heart block will may also benefit from temporary transvenous pacing. It should be noted, however, that the use of temporary pacing has never been statistically proven to improve prognosis.

○   **What is the most common sustained supraventricular arrhythmia in AMI?**

Sinus tachycardia. About one-third of patients will develop sinus tachycardia in the first days after acute AMI. The most common causes are anxiety, persistent pain, and left ventricular failure.

○   **What is the least common sustained supraventricular arrhythmia AMI?**

Atrial flutter, occurring in one to three percent.

○   **What is the most common sustained arrhythmia in AMI?**

Probably ventricular fibrillation, occurring in up to 10 percent of patients, and is seen more commonly in transmural infarction. The majority (60%) of VF events in AMI patients occur within 4 to 6 hours, and 80% by 12 hours. This "PrimaryVF" have been thought not to affect prognosis when treated rapidly, but some investigators have suggested this may indicate a worse prognosis.

○   **What is the best treatment for accelerated idioventricular rhythm (AIVR)?**

AIVR, characterized by a wide QRS rhythm with a rate faster than the atrial rate and less than 150/min, should not be treated, unless associated with a very significant drop in blood pressure. This rhythm is seen frequently in the early stages of AMI and occurs more often in patients with early reperfusion. However, it is neither sensitive nor specific enough to be considered a reliable marker for reperfusion.

○   **What is reperfusion injury?**

The acceleration of myocardial cell necrosis after reperfusion. It is characterized by rapid cellular swelling and wide spread architectural disruption. It is likely the acceleration of necrosis occurs in cells already destined to die, but it is possible that reperfusion may cause necrosis of reversibly injured myocardial cells as well.

○   **What factors predict development of pericarditis in AMI patients?**

Pericarditis usually occurs 1 day to 6 weeks after AMI. It is more common in males, q wave infarction and patients with congestive heart failure. Some reports suggest that pericarditis occurs in 10 to 20% of patients, but pericardial effusion without evidence of pericarditis is far more common.

○   **In AMI patients surviving their event, what is the most powerful predictor of long term survival?**

This is still debated, but the degree of increase in end systolic volume _may_ be the strongest. The extent of underlying left ventricular dysfunction (LVEF) and congestive heart failure are also strong predictors.

○   **How common is acute myocardial infarction (AMI)?**

It is estimated that one and a half million myocardial infarctions occur every year in the United States. Approximately one third of the patients with these events will die, with one half of deaths occurring prior to institution of medical therapy.

○   **What is the pathophysiology of acute MI?**

In general, acute occlusion secondary to thrombosis is considered the most common cause of AMI. Most transmural MI's are associated with complete obstruction, whereas non-transmural MI's may occur due to thrombosis alone, spasm with associated thrombosis, or, in significantly obstructed arteries, occur as a result of hypoxemia or hypotension.

○   **What is the most common cause of acute coronary thrombosis?**

Plaque disruption. Not all plaques have the same propensity to rupture. Characteristics rendering plaques "vulnerable" to disruption include: high lipid content, thin (as opposed to thick) fibrous cap, monocyte content, and shear forces present.

○   **What are the most common non-atherosclerotic causes of AMI?**

Embolization, arteritis, trauma, aortic or coronary dissection, and congenital anomalies.

○   **What is the most common cause of myocardial infarction in patients with angiographically normal coronary arteries?**

Approximately 6% of all MI patients, and as many as 25% of MI patients less than age 35 will have normal coronary anatomy by arteriography. Possible explanations for this include: oxygen demand-supply mismatch, prolonged hypotension, anatomic abnormalities of the coronary arteries, and hematologic disorders. It ha been theorized that coronary spasm and small vessel disease may also be possible causes.

○   **What are the most common metabolic disorders associated with increased risk of myocardial infarction?**

Hurler's disease, homocystinuria, Fabry's disease, amyloidosis, and pseudoxanthoma elasticum.

○   **What is the most common congenital anomaly associated with AMI?**

Anomalous origin of the left coronary artery from the pulmonary artery. If the left of right coronary artery originates from the contralateral aortic sinus, aberrant passage of the vessel between the aorta and the right ventricle outflow tract may result in MI, but more often results in sudden death.

○   **Describe the difference between "supply" and "demand" ischemia.**

Supply ischemia is due to occlusion or critical narrowing of the coronary artery, and it usually occurs in acute transmural MI. Demand ischemia is essentially due to a mismatch in oxygen supply and demand when coronary narrowing does not allow sufficient delivery of oxygen associated with the increased oxygen demand of an active myocardium. This more often occurs in unstable anginal syndromes and clinically defined non-Q wave MI.

○   **Why is the difference between supply and demand ischemia important?**

While the difference is a bit artificial, and both frequently occur together, the difference is important because different metabolic and mechanical changes occur in the myocardium depending upon the type of ischemia. The consequence of supply ischemia is the simultaneous development of cellular hypoxia and impaired washout of metabolites. As a result, the ischemia tissue becomes flaccid. In demand ischemia, while hypoxia also develops, washout of metabolites is relatively preserved, so contractility (which is related to a balance between calcium and inorganic phosphate and protons) is maintained.

○   **List the most common causes of myocardial oxygen supply-demand mismatch?**

Severe coronary artery disease, aortic stenosis, aortic insufficiency, carbon monoxide poisoning, thyrotoxicosis and prolonged hypotension.

○   **What are the phases of contraction abnormalities seen with acute cessation of blood flow to the myocardium?**

They occur sequentially and are generally categorized as: dysynchrony, hypokinesis, akinesis and dyskinesis.

○   **How much of the left ventricle needs to be involved before hemodynamic signs of left ventricular failure are present?**

Clinical congestive heart failure can occur with almost any left ventricular dysfunction. In AMI, hemodynamic evidence of left ventricular dysfunction occurs when 20 to 25% of the LV exhibits abnormal wall.

○   **What percentage of infarct-related coronary arteries, successfully opened with thrombolytic therapy, reocclude?**

15% of arteries, successfully opened, reocclude during the first few days following thrombolytic therapy.

○   **What is the mortality benefit from aspirin alone in acute myocardial infarction with thrombolytic therapy and in subsequent reinfarction?**

Aspirin reduced mortality from acute myocardial infarction by 23% and reduced non-fatal reinfarction by 49%. When used with thrombolytic therapy, there was a 40-50% reduction in mortality from acute myocardial infarction.

○   **A 47 year-old woman is admitted to you with substernal chest pressure for 1 hour. Serial ECG's and CK measurements confirm a non-Q wave anterior wall myocardial infarction. She has no arrhythmias, no evidence of heart failure and no recurrent chest pain while in the hospital. You**

discharge her on Diltiazem and aspirin on the fifth hospital day after she had a normal pre-discharge low-level treadmill exercise test. You schedule her for a symptom-limited treadmill test in two weeks. Three days after discharge, she reports a ten-minute episode of substernal chest pressure, while walking across the room, relieved with one sublingual nitroglycerin. What should you advise her to do?

Readmit her to the hospital, place her on intravenous heparin and nitroglycerin and perform cardiac catheterization with coronary angiography the following morning.

O   **A 56 year-old gentleman presents to your office three weeks after suffering an inferior wall myocardial infarction, treated successfully with r-TPA . He has non-insulin dependent diabetes mellitus. He denies any post-infarct symptoms. You supervise a symptom-limited treadmill exercise test which reveals 2 mm horizontal ST depression in the inferior and lateral leads after three minutes of exercise on Bruce protocol. On your recommendation, he undergoes a coronary angiogram and cardiac catheterization which reveals >70% stenosis of the proximal LAD, mid-RCA and first obtuse marginal branch of the circumflex. The LVEF on ventriculogram is 44%. What should you advise your patient at this time?**

Undergo 3-vessel coronary artery bypass graft surgery.

O   **A 60 year-old patient suffers an acute inferior myocardial infarction. Three hours after he arrives in the hospital, he develops ventricular fibrillation and is successfully defibrillated back to normal sinus rhythm within 30 seconds. He makes a full recovery and has no further post-MI complications. What does his ventricular fibrillation episode indicate with regard to his subsequent risk of sudden death?**

This episode has no bearing on his subsequent risk of sudden death. Ventricular fibrillation in the immediate setting of an acute myocardial infarction has no prognostic significance.

O   **What ECG changes arise in a true posterior infarction?**

Large R wave and ST depression in V1 and V2.

O   **What conduction defects commonly occur in an anterior wall MI?**

The dangerous kind. Damage to the conducting system results in a Mobitz II second or third degree AV block.

O   **How should PSVT be treated during an AMI?**

Vagal maneuvers, adenosine, or cardioversion. Stable patients may be able to tolerate negative inotropes, such as verapamil or even beta-blockers.

O   **A patient presents one day after discharge for an AMI with a new, harsh systolic murmur along the left sternal border and pulmonary edema. What is the diagnosis?**

Interventricular septal rupture. Diagnosis is confirmed with Swan-Ganz catheterization or echo. The treatment regime includes nitroprusside, for afterload reduction, and possibly an intra-aortic balloon pump followed by surgical repair.

O   **When does cardiac rupture usually occur in patients who have suffered acute MI's?**

Fifty percent arise within the first 5 days, and 90% occur within the first 14 days post-MI.

O   **Which type of infarct commonly leads to papillary muscle dysfunction?**

Inferior wall MI. Signs and symptoms include a mild transient systolic murmur and pulmonary edema.

O **A patient presents two weeks post AMI with chest pain, fever, and pleuropericarditis. A pleural effusion is detected by on CXR. What is the diagnosis?**

Dressler's (post-myocardial infarction) syndrome. This syndrome is caused by an immunologic reaction to myocardial antigens.

O **What percentage of patients over age 80 experience chest pain with an AMI?**

Only 50%. Twenty percent experience diaphoresis, stroke, syncope, and/or acute confusion.

O **Which type of thrombolytic agent is fibrin-specific?**

t-PA. This agent is a human protein with no antigenic properties.

O **What is unstable angina (UA)?**

In the absence of ECG or enzyme evidence of AMI, the term UA is usually applied in three historical circumstances: 1) New onset angina of Canadian class III or worse. 2) Angina at rest, as well as with minimal exertion. 3) More severe or prolonged angina in the context of a previous stable pain pattern. The more traditional definitions require one or more of these historical features with electrocardiographic changes, but many centers will classify patients as having unstable angina in the absence of ECG findings.

O **What is the primary pathophysiologic disturbance in UA?**

In general, patients presenting with UA tend to have more severe and/or extensive CAD, and a decrease in oxygen supply or an increase in demand may precipitate UA. Typically, reduction in oxygen supply is the primary problem and is usually the result of thrombosis (often with spontaneous recanalization) and less often the result of progression of atherosclerosis or vasoconstriction.

O **How does one treat unstable angina?**

UA, like AMI, is usually due to plaque rupture followed by platelet aggregation and thrombosis. Thus, the use of aspirin, heparin, or both is essential. Of note, while aspirin and heparin are both effective, there has not been definitive proof that either agent is better than the other, or that the combination is better than either agent alone. Use of nitroglycerin, beta-blockers, and calcium channel blockers are also standard therapy.

O **Are thrombolytic agents affective in non-Q wave MI?**

No, there is no evidence to support their use. In fact, some published data suggest that their use may be detrimental.

O **What is the prognosis of patients presenting with Q-wave MI complicated by acute mitral regurgitation?**

Prognosis is quite compromised with an approximate one-year survival of only 50%.

O **What is the best treatment of cardiogenic shock (SBP <90 and/or evidence of peripheral hypoperfusion)?**

The best treatment has not been established. Use of ionotropic agents and vasopressor agents is standard. The role of direct PTCA is still unresolved. Observational studies suggest a better outcome, but other studies have identified a selection bias in patients chosen for direct PTCA. Although survival remains dismal in patients presenting with shock, meta-analyses suggest there may be some benefit with administration of thrombolytic agents (particularly streptokinase).

ANGINA PECTORIS AND CORONARY ARTERY DISEASE

○ **What are the determinants of myocardial oxygen supply?**

The major determinants of myocardial oxygen supply are oxygen carrying capacity, coronary artery blood flow and vascular resistance. Vascular resistance is dependent by neural control, humoral factors, autoregulation, metabolic control, and extravascular compressive forces. Vascular resistance and diastolic coronary perfusion determine coronary blood flow.

○ **What are the determinants of myocardial oxygen consumption (or demand)?**

Heart rate, contractility and systolic wall tension are the major determinants. Other minor determinants include myocardial depolarization, metabolism of fatty acids, and direct metabolic effect of catecholamines.

○ **What is the clinical definition of angina pectoris?**

Angina pectoris is a chest discomfort, most commonly substernal, but occasionally left parasternal or left thoracic in location, lasting between 5 minutes and 30 minutes, described as "tightness", "squeezing", "constricting", "crushing", "vise-like", or "heaviness", often radiating to one or both shoulders and arms, occasionally radiating to the neck, jaw or epigastric area, most often occurring on exertion or excitement, but occasionally at rest, associated with diaphoresis, shortness of breath, palpitations, faintness, fatigue or nausea and relieved with nitroglycerin, or rest when precipitated by exercise.

○ **What are some other non-cardiac causes of angina-like chest pain?**

Esophageal spasm and motility disorders, gastroesophageal reflux disease, biliary colic, costochondral syndrome (Tietze's syndrome), and cervical radiculitis.

○ **What percentage of patients with chronic stable angina have a normal resting electrocardiogram?**

Approximately 50%.

○ **What is the most useful screening test employed in the diagnosis of coronary artery disease?**

The exercise electrocardiogram, or exercise treadmill test.

○ **What subset of patients is the exercise electrocardiogram most useful and reliable as a screening test for coronary artery disease?**

In patients whose resting electrocardiogram is normal, who are capable of achieving an adequate cardiac workload, and whose clinical symptoms and preponderance of risk factors for coronary artery disease suggest a moderate probability of having coronary artery disease.

○ **What specific abnormalities on the exercise electrocardiogram are strongly associated with multivessel coronary artery disease?**

Early onset of ST-segment depression, its long persistence following termination of exercise, downsloping or horizontal ST depression, and low work capacity or exercise duration are all associated strongly with multivessel disease.

O   **What is the positive predictive value of an exercise electrocardiogram that exhibits 1 mm downsloping or horizontal ST-segment depression in a patient <u>without</u> typical angina pectoris? 2 mm ST-segment depression?**

70% and 90%, respectively.

O   **What are the criteria for patients at high risk based on exercise electrocardiography?**

Greater than or equal to 2.0 mm ST-segment depression, greater than or equal to 1 mm ST-segment depression before the end of Stage I of Bruce protocol, ST-segment depression in multiple leads, ST-segment depression that lasts longer than 5 minutes during the recovery period, greater than 10 mmHg drop in systolic blood pressure during exercise, achievement of a cardiac workload less than 4 METS or a low exercise maximal heart rate, and significant ventricular arrhythmias, such as ventricular tachycardia.

O   **What are the criteria for patients at high risk based on exercise or pharmacological scintigraphy?**

Multiple perfusion defects (total plus reversible defects) in more than one vascular supply region (e.g., defects in coronary supply regions of the left anterior descending and left circumflex vessels), increased lung uptake of thallium or technetium (reflecting exercise-induced left ventricular dysfunction), and post-exercise transient left ventricular cavity dilatation.

O   **What is the likelihood of an asymptomatic patient with an abnormal exercise electrocardiogram and an abnormal exercise perfusion scintigraphy having coronary artery disease?**

Approximately 90%.

O   **What is the likelihood of patients with atypical chest pain having coronary artery disease if they have two abnormal noninvasive exercise or pharmacological tests?**

Over 95%.

O   **What is the likelihood of patients with atypical chest pain having coronary artery disease if they have a normal exercise electrocardiogram and myocardial perfusion study?**

Less than 5%.

O   **What percentage of patients with chronic stable angina, referred for coronary angiography, have no detectable critical coronary stenosis (> 70% luminal diameter narrowing)?**

15%.

O   **What percentage of patients with chronic stable angina, referred for coronary angiography, have left main coronary artery disease (> 50% luminal diameter narrowing)?**

5-10%.

O   **Which patients have more severe coronary artery disease as detected on coronary angiography - those with unheralded myocardial infarction or those with chronic stable angina?**

Patients with chronic stable angina. They tend to have more diseased vessels, more diffuse disease, more stenoses and more chronic occlusions.

❍   **In patients with single vessel disease and chronic stable angina, which regimen resulted in a greater number of patients free of angina at six months: PTCA or medical antianginal therapy?**

Those patients who underwent PTCA were more likely to be angina-free at six months.

❍   **In patients with multivessel coronary artery disease and moderate to severe LV systolic dysfunction (LVEF <35%), which strategy has the best long-term outcome: PTCA or CABG?**

CABG. Complete revascularization has a much better long-term outcome both for long-term survival and reduction of symptoms.

❍   **What are the determinants of an adverse prognosis in patients with coronary artery disease?**

Left ventricular dysfunction, large amount of myocardium in jeopardy, large amount of rest myocardial ischemia, multivessel coronary artery disease, serious ventricular arrhythmias, advanced age, history of congestive heart failure, diabetes mellitus, rapidly accelerating angina, presence of left ventricular hypertrophy, hyperlipidemia, abnormal resting electrocardiogram and presence of peripheral vascular disease.

❍   **What is the 5-year survival rate of patients with isolated right coronary artery disease medically treated?**

Approximately 96%.

❍   **What is the mortality of medically treated left main coronary artery disease?**

29% at 18 months, 39% at two years and 43% at 5 years for all patients with left main coronary artery stenosis greater than 50%. For patients with left main stenosis from 50-70%, the respective 1- and 3-year mortality rates are 9% and 34%. For patients with severe left main coronary artery disease (stenosis > 70%), the 1-year mortality is 28% and the 3-year mortality is 59%.

❍   **What percentage of asymptomatic middle-aged men have silent myocardial ischemia detected on exercise electrocardiography, radionuclide scanning or ambulatory electrocardiography?**

2.5%.

❍   **What time of the day is silent myocardial ischemia most frequent?**

Early morning, similar to the onset of acute myocardial infarction and unstable angina.

❍   **What is the most notable difference between silent myocardial ischemia and symptomatic myocardial ischemia?**

Silent myocardial ischemia tends to occur at heart rates that are lower than those associated with symptomatic myocardial ischemia.

❍   **What is the mortality in patients with silent myocardial ischemia?**

Mortality averages 2-3% per year. The presence of silent ischemia in patients with recent myocardial infarction or unstable angina significantly worsens the prognosis and should lead to an urgent and intense diagnostic and/or therapeutic intervention in these individuals.

❍   **What has happened to the overall mortality rate for patients with coronary artery disease?**

Decreased 56% since 1970.

○   **What are the factors that have contributed to the decline in mortality from coronary artery disease?**

Primary and secondary prevention of coronary artery disease, improved diagnosis, and most importantly, widespread effective medical and surgical therapy.

○   **What is the leading cause of death in women over age 50?**

Ischemic heart disease. It is responsible for 23% of all deaths in women, twice as many as cancer.

○   **Is sudden cardiac death more common in men or women?**

Men.

○   **What is the most common initial manifestation of coronary artery disease in women?**

Angina pectoris. A significantly higher percentage of men initially present with acute myocardial infarction or sudden death.

○   **Who has a better prognosis after the onset of angina pectoris or unrecognized myocardial infarction, men or women?**

Women.

○   **Who does has a better outcome with PTCA, men or women?**

Women. They have lower restenosis rates and better long-term survival following the procedure.

○   **Who has a better outcome with CABG, men or women?**

They have similar outcomes. Earlier studies suggested that women had a higher surgical mortality, a lower incidence of complete revascularization and a less favorable post-operative clinical response, but recent studies have shown that men and women have similar mortalities and similar outcomes.

○   **What is the most important prognostic factor in patients with chronic ischemic heart disease?**

Left ventricular function and severity of myocardial ischemia.

○   **What is the most common associated risk factor for coronary artery vasospasm (variant angina)?**

Cigarette smoking.

○   **T/F: The overwhelming majority of patients with variant angina will have an atherosclerotic plaque at the site of recurrent episodes of coronary arterial vasospasm.**

True.

○   **What other medical problems are patients with variant angina more prone to have?**

Migraine headaches, Raynaud's phenomenon and bronchial hyperreactivity.

○   **Do patients with variant angina have more episodes of coronary artery vasospasm and angina when treated with beta-blockers?**

No. While animal studies show that unopposed alpha-adrenergic vasoconstriction from beta-blocker therapy occurs in animal coronary anatomy, this has never been demonstrated in humans in any research trial. No evidence of coronary vasospasm detected on coronary angiography has ever been found with beta-blocker administration in any research study on humans.

O   **What is the most important factor in the dramatic improvement in survival in patients with variant angina?**

Widespread therapeutic use of calcium channel antagonists.

O   **What is Syndrome X?**

This syndrome is characterized by typical, usually exertional angina, a positive exercise electrocardiogram, coronary sinus lactate production during exercise or pacing and a normal coronary angiogram.

O   **What is the prognosis for patients with Syndrome X?**

Excellent. The incidence of sudden death and myocardial infarction is low.

O   **What are some of the physiologic and functional abnormalities of cardiac function and coronary blood flow in patients with Syndrome X?**

1.   Functionally abnormal coronary arteries with reduced vasodilatory responses to a variety of stimuli.
2.   Reduced myocardial blood flow following vasoconstrictive stimulation, e.g., ergonovine, cold pressors.
3.   Inadequate myocardial oxygenation during exercise.
4.   Abnormally reduced augmentation of systolic contraction.
5.   Reduced arteriolar vasodilatation.
6.   Abnormal left ventricular diastolic function
7.   Coronary artery endothelial cell dysfunction.

O   **What is the etiology of Syndrome X?**

Unknown.

O   **What is the most important and most dramatic secondary preventive measure in patients with coronary artery disease?**

Cessation of smoking. In general, there is a 40-50% reduction in risk of recurrent cardiac events or death in patients who quit smoking, compared to those who continue to smoke. The long-term risk for those who quit falls rapidly and approximates the risk of those who have never smoked by about 5 years after cessation.

O   **What other secondary prevention measures should be undertaken in patients with coronary artery disease?**

Successful lowering of serum lipids, augmentation of physical activity in the form of exercise, behavior modification and reduction of maladaptive behavior in response to stress, tighter control of blood glucose levels in patients with diabetes mellitus and successful control of blood pressure in patients with hypertension.

O   **What is the definition of unstable angina?**

Unstable angina is an intermediate coronary syndrome between angina pectoris and acute myocardial infarction. Its presence depends on one or more of the following three historical features: 1) crescendo angina (more severe, prolonged or frequent) superimposed on a pre-existing pattern or relatively stable, exertion-related angina pectoris, 2) angina pectoris of new onset (within one month) which is brought on by minimal exertion, or 3) angina pectoris at rest as well as minimal exertion. Variant angina, which is also characterized by angina at rest, has sometimes been considered to be a form of unstable angina, but it is pathogenically different from unstable angina.

○ What is the classification of unstable angina?

Class I –   New onset, severe or accelerated angina occurring within two months of presentation without rest pain. Also included in this class are patients whose angina is more frequent, severe, longer in duration or precipitated by substantially less exertion than previously.

Class II –   Patients with angina at rest during the preceding two months but not within the last 48 hours.

Class III-   Patients with rest angina at least once within the preceding 48 hours.

○ What are some of the clinical circumstances in which unstable angina occurs?

Secondary unstable angina refers to patients, usually with underlying obstructive CAD, in whom the imbalance between myocardial oxygen supply and demand causing the instability results from conditions that are extrinsic to the coronary vascular bed. This includes patients who have anemia or hypoxemia that cause reduced myocardial oxygen supply, as well as patients with fever, infection, aortic stenosis, uncontrolled hypertension, thyrotoxicosis, extreme emotional upset and tachyarrhythmias that cause increased myocardial oxygen demand.

Primary unstable angina, the most common form of unstable angina, occurs in the absence of an identifiable extracoronary condition and in patients who have not suffered an acute myocardial infarction within the preceding two weeks. Post-infarction unstable angina is present in patients who develop unstable angina within two weeks of a documented acute myocardial infarction; it occurs in approximately 20% of patients following infarction.

○ What is the etiology of primary unstable angina?

Atherosclerotic plaque rupture followed by platelet aggregation and thrombus formation. Aggregation of platelets and thrombus formation, usually superimposed on an atherosclerotic plaque, obstructs blood flow to the affected myocardium sufficiently long enough to cause ischemia and clinical symptoms, but not long enough to result in myocardial necrosis and infarction, as recanalization of the affected coronary artery occurs, usually within 20 minutes to one hour after the onset of plaque rupture. Unstable angina is often a precursor of acute myocardial infarction, and the two conditions share a common pathophysiologic link.

○ Among all patients with unstable angina, what percentage of patients have three-vessel coronary artery disease?

Approximately 40%.

○ Among all patients with unstable angina, what percentage of patients have left main coronary artery disease (> 50% stenosis)?

Approximately 20%.

○ Among all patients with unstable angina, what percentage of patients have no critical coronary obstruction on coronary angiogram?

Approximately 10%.

○ Among all patients with unstable angina, what percentage of patients have two-vessel coronary artery disease? Single-vessel CAD?

Approximately 20% have two-vessel CAD and 10% have single-vessel disease.

O   **What percentage of patients with unstable angina present with unstable angina as their <u>initial</u> manifestation of CAD?**

Approximately 50%.

O   **Of patients who present with unstable angina as their <u>initial</u> manifestation of CAD, what percentage of them have single-vessel CAD? Three-vessel disease?**

Approximately 50% have single-vessel disease (the majority have left anterior descending involvement) and less than 20% have three-vessel disease.

O   **What is the short-term prognosis of patients with unstable angina and no critical obstruction of a coronary artery on coronary angiogram (no intraluminal stenosis > 60%)?**

Excellent.

O   **What is the percentage of intracoronary thrombi found on coronary angiography in patients with unstable angina?**

50-70%.

O   **When a prior angiogram is available, the lesion responsible for an episode of unstable angina with documented ischemia is formerly greater than a 50% stenosis what percentage of the time? Formerly greater than 70% stenosis?**

Lesions responsible for acute ischemic episodes are formerly greater than 50% stenotic only 33-50% of the time and formerly greater than 70% less than 25% of the time.

O   **What percentage of patients with acute myocardial infarction have a prodrome of unstable angina shortly before infarction?**

Approximately 50%.

O   **What percentage of patients with unstable angina develop myocardial infarction in the short-term?**

Approximately 5%.

O   **What is the 5-year survival of patients with unstable angina rendered asymptomatic on medical therapy prior to discharge from the hospital who have a normal resting electrocardiogram and an exercise electrocardiogram negative for ischemia?**

Greater than 95%.

O   **Can patients with unstable angina, who have been stabilized and rendered asymptomatic on medical therapy prior to discharge from the hospital, be safely evaluated by exercise testing?**

Absolutely. However, coronary angiography is indicated for the vast majority of patients with unstable angina as the first diagnostic test, even in patients rendered asymptomatic by medical therapy.

O   **What factors portend a worse prognosis and signify a high-risk patient in those with unstable angina?**

Older patients, patients with continued rest pain despite medical therapy, and patients with thrombi, complex coronary morphology or multivessel disease on coronary angiography. Patients who have ischemia detected on ambulatory electrocardiographic monitoring and those with significant ST-T wave abnormalities at presentation are also at higher risk and tend to have an unfavorable outcome.

○   **What is the most useful diagnostic test in the evaluation of patients with unstable angina?**

Coronary angiography.

○   **What is the hallmark of drug therapy for patients admitted with unstable angina?**

Intravenous low molecular-weight heparin and at least 81 mg of aspirin daily. Intravenous nitroglycerin is strongly recommended for patients with Class II or Class III unstable angina, but one must keep in mind to increase the dose of intravenous heparin during intravenous nitroglycerin administration as nitroglycerin reduces the efficacy of heparin.

○   **What is the role of thrombolytic therapy in unstable angina?**

None. To date, no clinical trial has shown any benefit of thrombolytic therapy, presumably because thombi in unstable angina tend to be platelet-rich, not fibrin-rich, and thus resistant to thrombolytic therapy.

○   **What are some other highly efficacious drug therapies in patients with unstable angina?**

Beta-blockers have been shown to be highly effective in reducing the frequency and duration of both symptomatic and silent myocardial ischemic episodes. Calcium channel antagonists, while not as efficacious as beta-blockers in reducing myocardial oxygen demand, are highly effective in reducing symptoms and ischemic episodes, but should not be used as monotherapy. In fact, monotherapy with nifedipine in unstable angina is associated with an increase in non-fatal myocardial infarctions within the first 48 hours after initiation of therapy.

○   **What percentage of patients with unstable angina are refractory to maximal medical therapy?**

Approximately 9%. These patients are quite vulnerable to adverse results during PTCA and CABG and should be strongly considered for intra-aortic balloon counterpulsation prior to any further intervention.

○   **A 66 year-old gentleman with unstable angina is referred to you for evaluation. He has been on intravenous heparin, nitroglycerin and aspirin for two days in the ICU and has had no further episodes of chest pain or ischemic episodes on ECG. You perform coronary angiography on him and find a 75% stenosis with an irregular-shaped thrombus in the mid-LAD. What should you do next?**

The presence of a coronary thrombus is associated with lower success rates for PTCA and higher complication rates. PTCA performed in patients more than 2 weeks after the onset of unstable angina has a higher success rate and a lower complication rate than when it is performed within the first two weeks. It is recommended that he continue on intravenous heparin for at least 2-3 more days, along with aspirin, and be scheduled for elective PTCA in about 3 weeks, provided he has no further episodes of unstable angina. Intracoronary thrombolytic therapy is also a reasonable consideration in selected patients in order to dissolve the thrombus.

○   **What is the risk of abrupt coronary closure during or within 24 hours after a PTCA in a patient with an intracoronary thrombus?**

2-9 times higher than when performed in the absence of an intracoronary thrombus.

○   **What is the role of CABG in patients with unstable angina?**

CABG is reserved for patients who fail medical therapy and who are not amenable to PTCA or for patients with three-vessel CAD with reduced left ventricular function or left main coronary artery disease (>50% stenosis).

○ **What is the role of PTCA in unstable angina?**

In patients refractory to medical therapy with single-vessel or two-vessel disease in whom the culprit lesion has not been stabilized with maximal medical therapy.

○ **What is the 1-year incidence of myocardial infarction in patients with unstable angina who received medical therapy without revascularization?**

10-27%. The incidence of myocardial infarction within one month of hospitalization is 8-13%.

○ **What is the 1-year mortality of patients with unstable angina who received medical therapy without revascularization?**

9-19%. The incidence of death is 4% in the first month after hospitalization.

○ **What factors adversely affect the outcome of patients with unstable angina?**

Persistence of pain in the hospital, previous chronic angina and older age.

○ **What is the strategy for managing patients with unstable angina?**

1. All patients should receive immediate medical therapy with an eye to stabilization.
2. Patients who remain unstable and those deemed candidates for invasive management should
3. be referred for cardiac catheterization within 48 hours of presentation, provided there are no contraindications to invasive therapy.
4. Patients who stabilize easily and who are not at high risk for complications, and those patients who prefer continued medical management, or those who are not candidates for invasive therapy because of contraindications should continue on intensive medical therapy.
5. Patients should be strongly considered for cardiac catheterization if they have one or more of the following high-risk indicators: prior revascularization, associated congestive heart failure or depressed LVEF (< 50%) by non-invasive study, malignant ventricular arrhythmias, persistent or recurrent pain/ischemia, and/or a functional study indicating a high risk.

○ **What percentage of patients who have sudden cardiac death have a prior history or angina, myocardial infarction or congestive heart failure?**

50%.

○ **In patients with sudden cardiac death, what percentage of patients are found to have a coronary thrombus on autopsy?**

30-75%. It is most commonly found in patients with single-vessel CAD and those with acute myocardial infarction or recent unstable angina. It is less common in patients with previous myocardial infarction or three-vessel CAD.

○ **What medical regimen can one use in patients with unstable angina who have a contraindication or a major complication to intravenous heparin?**

Ticlopidine, at a dose of 250 mg twice daily, or clopidogrel at 75 mg per day are very suitable alternatives to heparin. Furthermore, unlike intravenous heparin, they can be feasibly continued in the outpatient setting.

O   **Among survivors of sudden cardiac death without myocardial infarction, which group of patients are more likely to have complex coronary atherosclerotic lesions: those with inducible ventricular tachycardia or those without inducible ventricular tachycardia on electrophysiology testing?**

Those patients without inducible ventricular tachycardia, suggesting those survivors of sudden cardiac death without inducible ventricular tachycardia on electrophysiology testing had ischemia as their precipitating event, while those who had inducible ventricular tachycardia had an arrhythmic etiology of their sudden cardiac death episode.

O   **A 51 year-old female school teacher suffers an inferior myocardial infarction. Her hospital course is uncomplicated. On day 5 following her myocardial infarction, she undergoes a submaximal exercise treadmill test. She develops 2.5 mm ST depression in the inferior and lateral leads. What is the best immediate intervention in this patient?**

Cardiac catheterization with coronary angiography.

O   **A 45 year-old menstruating female smoker comes to your office with complaints of having been awakened from sleep by substernal chest discomfort associated with palpitations. A 24-hour ambulatory ECG reveals an episode of ST-segment elevation occurring simultaneously with the chest discomfort. What is her coronary angiogram likely to show?**

Luminal irregularities in an epicardial segment of a coronary artery, but no critical stenosis. In other words, early coronary artery disease.

O   **A 59 year-old man comes to you for a second opinion. He has been advised to undergo cardiac catheterization. He sustained an anterior wall myocardial infarction 10 weeks ago, but is currently asymptomatic. He is only on aspirin. A technetium-99m sestamibi exercise test (Bruce protocol) demonstrates a fixed anterior wall defect with minimal peri-infarct redistribution. The LVEF is 52%. The patient exercises for 11.5 minutes and stops secondary to fatigue. What would you recommend this patient to do?**

Start beta-blocker therapy and recommend against cardiac catheterization. His prognosis is good and coronary angiography will add very little to his therapeutic management.

O   **An 81 year-old gentleman, formerly vigorous and active, reports frequent episodes of exertional angina pectoris, relieved by rest and sublingual nitroglycerin. His resting pulse is 40/min; the resting ECG is normal except for marked sinus bradycardia and first degree AV block (PR interval = .26 seconds). The patient's blood pressure is 125/72 mmHg and his serum cholesterol is 235 mg/dl. What would be the most appropriate strategy in this patient?**

Coronary angiography. This patient undoubtedly has coronary artery disease that is causing symptoms and conduction system disease. A pacemaker is not indicated as he has not had syncope, dizziness or fatigue. Coronary angiography should be performed with an eye toward revascularization. Cholesterol-lowering therapy would be of little help in this individual.

O   **A 49 year-old policeman develops 3 mm ST-segment elevation in leads I, aVL and V6 during an exercise electrocardiogram performed because of new-onset exertional dyspnea. Coronary angiography demonstrates the following: a 30% stenosis in the mid-left anterior descending coronary artery, two sequential 40% distal stenoses in the right coronary artery and a 90% stenosis in the proximal left circumflex coronary artery. What is the best therapeutic option for this patient?**

PTCA of the left circumflex artery. This is preferable to medical therapy and his coronary disease is not severe enough to warrant coronary bypass surgery.

○   A 41 year-old male has presented to the emergency department, reporting that he had an uncomfortable feeling in his upper chest and left shoulder 10 days ago. He recently had some highly flavored food and felt better after taking an antacid. The chest and shoulder discomfort recurred spontaneously at his desk 3 days ago, lasting for 10 minutes, and it recurred this evening, lasting 10-15 minutes. It resolved while he drove himself to the hospital. He is presently pain free and his ECG is normal. Blood pressure was 150/95 mmHg, his exam and lab work are normal, and he wants to go home, stating that he has an important business meeting in a distant city in 2 days. The emergency department physician has diagnosed gastroesophageal reflux and wants you to approve his discharge. The patient is a smoker and has a family history of CAD. What is the best advice you can give?

Admit the patient for 23-hour observation and plan coronary angiography the following morning.

○   A 55 year-old woman complains of exertional substernal chest discomfort. The patient is a non-smoker, her blood pressure is 110/70 mmHg and her serum cholesterol is 200 mg/dl. A treadmill exercise test demonstrates 3 mm ST-segment depression in leads II, III, aVF, and V5-6. A coronary angiogram reveals normal coronary arteries. Which pharmacologic agent(s) would be most beneficial in this patient?

Calcium channel antagonists, nitrates and imipramine would all be efficacious in this patient.

○   A 77 year-old man presents complaining of chest pain. He states that he was playing racquet-ball, and slipped and hit his head on the wall. After this he noted the onset of chest pain radiating to the arm. A hot shower did not relieve his symptoms. He notes that he has continued to have dull ache in his chest. He also reports an episode of diaphoresis after the shower and mild nausea. ECG reveals acute anterior wall MI. What would you do to treat him?

Administer aspirin immediately. The choice for additional therapy is complicated by the presence of head trauma. In the proper setting, direct PTCA is the treatment of choice, since it produces higher TIMI-3 flow rates and defines the coronary anatomy, with a lower stroke risk. The benefits of direct PTCA over thrombolytic therapy, while still debated, require a high operator volume and access to a lab within 60-90 minutes. If direct PTCA is not available for this patient, the decision to give thrombolytic therapy is a difficult one.

HEART FAILURE AND CARDIOMYOPATHY

○ **What is "physiologic" hypertrophy?**

An adaptive change in left ventricular wall thickness as a response to isotonic or isometric exercise. Isotonic exercise in athletes causes eccentric or volume dependent hypertrophy, and reverses with discontinuance of training. In contrast, isometric exercise, such as weight lifting, causes concentric hypertrophy, analogous to hypertension, resulting from intermittent increases in afterload. This, too, may demonstrate regression when training has stopped.

○ **What pathologic disorders result in concentric left ventricular hypertrophy?**

Hypertension and aortic stenosis are the most common. Other causes include coronary artery disease, myocardial infiltrative disorders, such as amyloidosis, pheochromocytoma, coarctation of the aorta, diabetes mellitus, and hypertrophic cardiomyopathy.

○ **What disorders result in eccentric left ventricular hypertrophy?**

Regurgitant valvular heart disease and obesity are the two most common causes. Eccentric left ventricular hypertrophy occurs as a response to volume overload and manifests as increased left ventricular wall thickness and chamber volume.

○ **What are the major complications of left ventricular aneurysms?**

LV thrombus formation (with the subsequent risk of thromboembolic events), CHF, and ventricular arrhythmias.

○ **A 60 year-old man with a recent syncopal episode is hospitalized with congestive heart failure and chest pain. His BP is 165/85 mm Hg, his pulse is 85/min and there is a grade III/VI harsh systolic murmur at the apex and aortic area. An echocardiogram reveals a disproportionately thickened septum and anterior systolic motion of the mitral valve. What is this patient's diagnosis and what physical findings would most likely be present?**

Obstructive hypertrophic cardiomyopathy (IHSS). The murmur typically decreases with handgrip and Valsalva, and increases with vasodilators, standing, nitroglycerin, diuretics and digoxin. Mitral regurgitation is frequent as a result of anterior systolic motion of the mitral valve. Congestive heart failure is present because of diastolic dysfunction; thus an S4 gallop is common.

○ **What is the most common primary malignant cardiac neoplasm?**

Sarcoma.

○ **What is the most common benign cardiac tumor?**

Myxoma.

○ **What is the definitive treatment of an atrial myxoma?**

Surgical excision. The risk for embolization is very high and emergent surgical excision is warranted.

O   **Which are more common: left atrial myxomas or right atrial myxomas?**

Right atrial myxomas.

O   **Aside from the high risk of embolization, what are the non-embolic risks of atrial myxomas?**

They act as a ball-valve obstruction to flow across either the tricuspid valve or mitral valve and can cause markedly reduced ventricular filling with resultant reduction in cardiac output and progressive heart failure. They can also cause tricuspid or mitral valve incompetence and lead to significant insufficiency and resultant heart failure.

O   **Which is the most common type of cardiomyopathy?**

Dilated cardiomyopathy. This condition is induced by progression of myocarditis, alcohol, adriamycin, diabetes mellitus, pheochromocytoma, thiamine deficiency, thyroid disease, and valvular heart disease. The other types of cardiomyopathies are hypertrophic and restrictive.

O   **What is the most common discharge diagnosis in patients over 65?**

CHF.

O   **Which is the most common type of cardiac failure, high or low output?**

Low output failure. Reduced stroke volume, lowered pulse pressure, and peripheral vasoconstriction are all signs of low output failure.

O   **What is the most common cause of low output heart failure in the world?**

Chagas' disease. In addition to heart failure, patients present with prolonged fever, hepatosplenomegaly, megaesophagus, megacolon, edema, and lymphadenopathy. This disease is most prevalent in Latin America.

O   **What is the most common cause of low output heart failure in the US?**

CAD. Other causes include congenital heart disease, cor pulmonale, dilated cardiomyopathy, hypertension, hypertrophic cardiomyopathy, infection, toxins, and valvular heart disease.

O   **What is the comparative mortality rates from CHF between the sexes?**

Women fair slightly better. The 5-year mortality rate for a female with CHF is 45%, as compared to 60% for males. The majority of deaths from CHF result from ventricular arrhythmias.

O   **Describe the 3 stages of CXR findings in CHF.**

Stage I: Pulmonary arterial wedge pressure (PAWP) of 12 to 18 mm Hg. Blood flow increases in the upper lung fields (cephalization of pulmonary vessels).

Stage II: PAWP of 18 to 25 mm Hg. Interstitial edema is evident with blurred edges of blood vessels and Kerley B lines.

Stage III: PAWP > 25 mm Hg. Fluid exudes into alveoli with the generation of the classic butterfly pattern of perihilar infiltrates.

O   **Rales are present on exam in a 50 year-old man with recent anterior wall MI. What can you say about the pulmonary artery occlusion ("wedge") pressure?**

It is likely above 20 to 25 mm Hg.

O   **A 30 year-old woman with long-standing idiopathic cardiomyopathy has faint basilar crackles on lung exam. What would you expect her pulmonary wedge pressure to be?**

In chronic heart failure, patients may have elevated wedge pressures (a reflection of elevated left ventricular end diastolic pressure) greater than 30mm Hg with only minor findings on lung exam. This is likely due to increased pulmonary lymphatic drainage.

O   **Can the chest radiograph show signs of systolic heart failure when the physical exam is negative?**

Rales on exam develop when there is extravasated fluid within the alveoli. The first site fluid accumulates in hydrostatic pulmonary edema is the interstitial space that surrounds blood vessels and bronchi. This interstitial fluid is visible on X-rays before the exam becomes positive.

O   **A 65 year-old man 3 days post an uncomplicated inferior wall MI is noted to have basilar crackles on lung exam that mostly clear with coughing. His creatinine is 2.1, and he weighs 75 kg. Approximately how much furosemide should you administer for adequate diuresis?**

Probably none. In the proper clinical context, rales are obviously a useful sign of heart failure, even in its incipient stage. Since most ICU patients are bed-bound and will experience atelectasis of dependent lung tissue, the patient should be reexamined after a few vigorous coughs and gentle pulmonary toilet. Very often rales and diuretics will soon disappear from the bedside.

O   **You suspect severe LV systolic dysfunction in a new ICU admission. A pulmonary artery catheter is placed. However, your pressure transducer is malfunctioning and your cardiac output machine is broken. What *laboratory test* will confirm your suspicions?**

Measurement of the mixed venous saturation is an extremely useful measure of low-output state in heart failure. With reduced systolic function, peripheral tissues will extract more oxygen; this will reduce the mixed venous oxygen saturation, often dramatically.

O   **A 65 year-old man complains of fatigue and shortness of breath. Exam: rales and edema; a displaced PMI with a systolic murmur at the left sternal border radiating to the aortic area, and a holosystolic murmur at the apex radiating to the axilla. Echo: low normal LV function, aortic valve sclerosis with a peak gradient on continuos wave Doppler study of 40 mm Hg. Color Doppler not performed. Pulmonary artery catheter findings: cardiac output 2.4; mixed venous oxygen saturation: 45% (Normal: (65%). How do you explain the patient's low-output state by pulmonary artery catheterization, given preserved LV function and non-critical AS on echocardiogram?**

This patient emphasizes the importance of the mixed venous oxygen saturation: this low number, suggesting increased extraction of oxygen from the periphery and a low output state, appears to contradict the echo data. However, the patient has mitral regurgitation (MR) on exam, the severity of which was not reported on echo. A repeat study demonstrated severe MR, and revealed an important contributing factor to the patient's low output state.

O   **A 70 year-old admitted four days ago with inferior wall MI is short of breath. A recent echocardiogram reports (but does not grade the severity of) mitral regurgitation (MR). You insert a pulmonary artery catheter and note a giant V wave on wedge tracing. Can you correlate the height of the V wave with the degree of MR?**

Beware! Giant V waves may not even *indicate* MR! V wave size is related to the volume of blood entering the left atrium (as it is reflected back in the wedge tracing) and also to left atrial compliance. Sever MR with a large, distended left atrium may not exhibit a giant V wave. Alternatively, a hypervolemic patient with no MR may acutely distend a normal-sized LA and demonstrate giant V waves. The present patient actually has a ventricular septa defect (VSD) as a complication of MI; increased pulmonary blood flow through the VSD produced a "hypervolemic" state, giant V waves, and CHF.

○   **What is preload?**

The wall stress that the ventricle (LV) sees at the end of diastole, which is determined by venous return. In the normal heart, when preload increases, the LV distends, the resting length of the sarcomere increases, and the LV can generate greater pressures more rapidly, augmenting stroke volume.

○   **What is afterload?**

The load against which the LV must contract as systole begins—that is, the pressure the LV must generate to open the aortic valve and then eject blood.

○   **What is the law of Laplace?**

A simplified equation that describes the factors governing wall stress in a chamber (i.e., the LV). According to Laplace, wall stress equals the pressure within a chamber multiplied by the radius of the chamber, divided by twice the chamber's wall thickness (pressure x radius / 2 x wall thickness). If wall stress increases, the LV must work harder, and myocardial oxygen uptake (and demand) increase.

○   **How many Gatorade-guzzling weight lifters with reduced left ventricular systolic function and symptoms of heart failure does it take to lift Dr. Laplace?**

Clean-and-jerking physiologists should be avoided in patients with systolic heart failure. A more common clinical scenario would be that of an infected, intubated, agitated patient with a history of old anterior wall MI and ejection fraction of 20%, on norepinephrine and intravenous fluid infusion for hypotension, with a blood pressure of 160/100, who is "bucking the ventilator". Fluid infusion is increasing venous return and LV preload—possibly to inappropriate pressure levels. The patient's scarred LV is thinned (decreased wall thickness) and dilated (increased radius) and his agitation and pressors are raising his blood pressure inappropriately (increased chamber pressure from afterload). This patient's wall stress is dramatically increased, and his compromised myocardial reserve puts him at great risk for hemodynamic decompensation.

○   **You are asked to evaluate hypotension in an elderly woman. On evaluation, the patient complains of chest pain. She is diaphoretic; her lips are dusky; her radial pulse is faint and slow. Jugular venous distension is present, but the lung fields are clear. Glancing at her bedside monitor, you conclude that her central venous line has migrated distally, since there is a right ventricular pressure tracing. What's going on?**

The patient is having a right ventricular infarction with hypotension secondary to *right* ventricular failure. The physical exam findings are classic. The central line has not migrated, but is showing a characteristic "ventricularized" tracing.

○   **Sustained ventricular tachycardia is well controlled in a 55 year-old man post non-Q wave MI with lidocaine 2 microgram/ml. He has a known history of ischemic cardiomyopathy. Day 3 of his admission, his speech becomes slurred, he is lethargic, and, when aroused, becomes very agitated. What should you do?**

This patient has classic findings of lidocaine toxicity, and you should strongly consider stopping this drug. Elderly patients, patients with heart failure, and those with hepatic insufficiency are especially at risk.

○   **An elderly man with progressive symptoms of shortness of breath is intubated for respiratory failure. He has a 100 pack-year smoking history. On exam, he is agitated and "bucking the vent". Breath sounds are coarse throughout, heart sounds faint. External jugular veins are prominently** distended. His liver edge is palpable; his extremities are dusky, with lower extremity pitting edema. EKG shows sinus tachycardia and poor R wave progression. The BUN/creatinine ratio is elevated. You have concluded that the patient has systolic heart failure. What is your next step?

Reconsider your diagnosis! The ICU is fraught with physical exam pitfalls. JVD may be difficult to interpret—especially in a patient who is increasing his intrathoracic pressure by breathing out of synch with the ventilator. Patients with COPD can have dusky extremities; they may have coarse breath sounds throughout their lung fields; pulmonary hypertension and RV dysfunction may lead to peripheral edema; diaphragmatic or abdominal viscera displacement may alter the axis of the hear and affect EKG interpretation. Under such circumstances, a bedside echo may be very helpful.

O   **A 60 year-old man with a recent syncopal episode is hospitalized with congestive heart failure and chest pain. His BP is 165/85 mm Hg, his pulse is 85/min and there is a grade III/VI harsh systolic murmur at the apex and aortic area. An echocardiogram reveals a disproportionately thickened septum and anterior systolic motion of the mitral valve. What is this patient's diagnosis and what physical findings would most likely be present?**

Obstructive hypertrophic cardiomyopathy (IHSS). The murmur typically decreases with handgrip and Valsalva, and increases with vasodilators, standing, nitroglycerin, diuretics and digoxin. Mitral regurgitation is frequent as a result of anterior systolic motion of the mitral valve. Congestive heart failure is present because of diastolic dysfunction; thus an S4 gallop is common.

O   **A patient presents with a history of episodic elevations in BP. She complains of headache, diarrhea, and skin flushing. What is the likely diagnosis?**

Pheochromocytoma.

O   **What are the acute hemodynamic effects of furosemide administration?**

Furosemide increases venous capacitance and lowers wedge pressure within minutes of IV bolus infusion – a notable effect in CHF exacerbations.

O   **A 72 year-old woman admitted to the ICU with pulmonary edema is much improved after overnight diuresis. Soon after you note that she is 4 liters negative in fluid balance, she develops polymorphic VT requiring cardioversion. Her regular medications include 80 mg bid of furosemide. What is a likely etiology?**

Beware of electrolyte abnormalities, especially hypokalemia, inducing Torsade de Pointes in CHF patients after vigorous diuresis – especially in patients on chronic diuretics.

O   **You correct the electrolyte imbalances in the above patient, and she is carefully diuresed another 2 liters. Vital signs are stable, with BP 120/80, HR 80. Echo reveals an LVEF of 35% and you initiate Captopril 25 mg every eight hours. Two hours later, the patient complains of dizziness; BP is 80/60, HR is 100. What happened?**

ACE inhibitors can have a profound first dose effect and lead to symptomatic hypotension, especially in patients, like this one, who have been aggressively diuresed. The peak effect with a short acting agent such as Captopril will occur 1 to 2 hours after the initial dose. Careful volume expansion usually reverses this effect. It's best to initiate ACE therapy with a low dose of short acting drug (i.e., captopril 6.25 mg) especially in acutely ill patients.

O   **A 65 year-old man with known severe hypertension, past CHF and COPD is intubated for acute pulmonary edema and suspected pneumonia. PB is 190/110; 92 saturation is 94% on 60% O_2. You successfully lower his blood pressure to 140/80 with intravenous sodium nitroprusside. However, the patient develops chest pressure and you note that his O_2 saturation is now 86%. What happened?**

Two effects of nitroprusside are likely culprits. Nonselective dilation of the pulmonary arteriolar bed can worsen ventilation-perfusion mismatch, especially in patients with COPD or pneumonia, and cause desaturation. "Coronary steal" (reduced perfusion to coronary arteries with fixed obstruction in the setting of arteriolar dilation by nitroprusside) may lead to ischemia and chest pain.

○ **A patient presents with systolic left ventricular failure. QRS voltage is diffusely decreased on EKG. On echocardiogram, LV wall thickness is preserved, but has a "speckled" appearance. What diagnosis should you consider?**

Amyloidosis.

○ **You are asked to assist in the management of a patient with acute CHF that is refractory to diuretic therapy. You are informed that a total of 120 mg of furosemide has been administered. What important question must you ask?**

Diuretics often require the administration of a threshold dose to be effective. The question you should ask is: "How was the furosemide administered"? An initial dose of 40 mg, followed by a second dose of 80 mg (double the dose) would be appropriate. Often the answer will be that three doses of furosemide, 40 mg each, were administered.

○ **A 70 year-old man with systolic heart failure is refractory to appropriately administered escalating doses of furosemide. Name an option to treat his diuretic resistance.**

Loop diuretics are the only class of diuretics effective as single agents in moderate to sever CHF. Often, adding a second agent with a different site of action in the nephron – i.e., a thiazide diuretic that prevents fluid resorption at a site distal to the loop of Henle – will enhance diuresis.

○ **Name two important complications of the above therapy.**

Profound intravascular volume and potassium depletion.

○ **Despite appropriate medical therapy, including combination diuretics, a 75 year-old woman with reduced systolic function in acute pulmonary edema remains oliguric. What *"mechanical"* intervention may increase her urine output?**

Intubation or CPAP, if she can tolerate it. A large portion of her (already decreased) cardiac out is going to her overworked diaphragm. Decreasing her work of breathing will allow better perfusion of her kidneys, and can lead to dramatic diuresis.

○ **The above patient has a 2.5 liter diuresis after intubation. She is placed on a CMV mode with 10 of PEEP. The next morning, her lungs are clear. You attempt a T-piece wean, but not rales throughout both lung fields within minutes. What are three possible explanations?**

1) You've increased her work of breathing prematurely (i.e., before maximizing other therapies). 2) Coronary artery disease with concomitant ischemia may be contributing. 3) You've abruptly withdrawn potent cardiopulmonary effects of positive pressure ventilation. By increasing intrathoracic pressure, CMV and PEEP decrease the pressure gradient for venous blood flow from the great vessels to the right atrium, thereby decreasing preload; positive pressure against the heart can also have afterload reducing effects.

○ **A 55 year-old man presents with progressive dyspnea and rales on exam. Past medical history reveals no significant cardiac risk factors, no alcohol or drug use; it is significant only for a stab would to the right groin many years ago. On examination of the lower extremities, there is unilateral warmth and edema of the right leg. You note a continuous murmur over the femoral artery. What type of heart failure does the patient have?**

The exam and history are consistent with an acquired arteriovenous fistula leading to high-output heart failure.

O   **You are called to the bedside of a 65 year-old woman with an EF of 20% to assess hypotension. She presented with pulmonary edema, but was effectively diuresed and started on therapy with ACE inhibitors, digoxin and lasix. BP is 80/60, HR is 80, RR is 12. Exam: no JVD, clear lungs, no murmurs or gallops, no peripheral edema. Urine output is 45 cc/hour. Should you decrease her ACE inhibitor, diuretic or both?**

Neither. Despite the patient's low blood pressure, there is no evidence of organ hypoperfusion.

O   **Describe the typical findings for cardiac output, arterial-mixed venous oxygen difference and systemic vascular resistance in systolic heart failure.**

Cardiac output is low; due to increased extraction of oxygen from the periphery, arterial-mixed venous oxygen difference is increased; systemic vascular resistance is increased (the periphery is "clamped down").

O   **A 27 year-old man with a past history of receiving chemotherapy for a hematologic malignancy presents with worsening dyspnea on exertion for several months. Exam reveals JVD and rales throughout both lung fields. X-ray of the chest demonstrates cardiomegaly. Echocardiogram shows four-chamber dilation with severely reduced LV function. What chemotherapeutic agent might the patient have received?**

Doxorubicin, which can present with cardiomyopathy even years after its initial administration.

O   **What are two reasons why dobutamine, in general, is a superior inotrope in heart failure to dopamine?**

1. Dobutamine acts as a peripheral dilator and reduces systemic vascular resistance, whereas dopamine, even at intermediate infusion rates, may cause peripheral vasoconstriction. 2. Tachycardia and arrhythmias tend to occur more frequently with dopamine than dobutamine.

O   **A 50 year-old man presents with pulmonary edema. Past medical history is significant only for chest pain on exertion. Echo reveals LV hypokinesis with an LVEF of 30%. He receives appropriate diuresis and therapy with ACE inhibitors and digoxin. What additional work up would be appropriate?**

The patient requires an evaluation for ischemic heart disease as a possible etiology not just of his chest pain but also his decreased LV function. In the setting of chest pain, cardiac catheterization is an appropriate next step.

O   **Name an etiology for the side effect of cough in ACE inhibitor administration.**

Inhibition of bradykinin metabolism.

O   **How do you adjust the dose of ACE inhibitor to prevent the development of ACE related cough in the asthmatic patient?**

Patients with underlying lung disease or asthma are not at risk for developing ACE inhibitor-induced cough, which develops in up to 5% of patients on chronic therapy.

O   **What is the role of digoxin in reducing mortality in systolic heart failure?**

In patients receiving ACE inhibitors and diuretics, the addition of digoxin reduces the number of hospitalizations for heart failure; it has not clearly been shown to reduce mortality.

○   **On average, how long does a patient with severe aortic stenosis have to live after developing symptoms of heart failure?**

Two years.

○   **An 80 year-old woman with a history of pulmonary edema once again presents in heart failure. Past admissions have noted a loud, harsh systolic radiating to the base. You note the murmur, but it is barely audible on your exam. What cardiac lesion should you suspect?**

Episodes of recurrent CHF in an elderly person should prompt evaluation for occult aortic stenosis. Worsening heart function can lead to a diminished intensity of the murmur.

○   **You place a pulmonary artery catheter in a severely malnourished alcoholic with edema on physical exam and cardiomegaly on X-ray. Findings include an elevated cardiac output and a decreased arterial-mixed venous oxygen difference and systemic vascular resistance. What diagnosis should you consider?**

These are classic hemodynamic findings in beriberi heart disease (thiamine deficiency).

○   **An 80 year-old man intubated for systolic heart failure has diuresed well acutely, but still has CHF on X-ray and an elevated wedge pressure of 22 mg Hg. Vitals: BP is 100/75, HR is 85, FiO_2 is 50% and O_2 Sat is 93%. To improve the O_2 sat and wedge pressure and treat the X-ray, your intern adds 15 mm Hg of PEEP ("expanding collapsed alveoli") and administers a large dose of furosemide. 1 liter of diuresis later, the patient's SBP is 85, HR is 120, and wedge is 24 mm Hg! As you grab the next IV dose of furosemide from your intern's sweaty little hand, what pathophysiological thoughts run through your head?**

1) 22 mg Hg may represent an "adequate" filling pressure in the setting of reduced LV function. 2) X-ray findings may lag behind clinical improvement. 3) By increasing intrathoracic pressures, PEEP may spuriously elevate wedge pressure and not be an accurate measure of LV filling pressures – i.e., this patient may be relatively "dry" (increased heart rate, low blood pressure) despite a higher wedge pressure.

○   **Two weeks ago you doubled the diuretic dose of an 80 year-old woman receiving standard therapy for systolic heart failure. She is subsequently admitted to the ICU with confusion, nausea and vomiting and third-degree heart block. What important drug level should you check?**

Serum digoxin. Worsening renal insufficiency, in this case induced by increasing diuretics, can significantly prolong the half-life of digoxin. This is the most common cause of toxicity in chronic digoxin therapy.

○   **A 25 year-old woman presents with symptoms of heart failure and sinus tachycardia on EKG. Echo reveals a dilated LV and severely reduced systolic function. Despite appropriate therapy, including ace-inhibitors, diuretics and digoxin, the patient remains tachycardic. Elaborate on chickens and eggs.**

"Which came first, the chicken or the egg?" is an important pearl when cardiomyopathy appears to be related to an inappropriately fast heart rate. Various supraventricular tachycardias (atrial, inappropriate sinus) can lead to a tachycardia-induced cardiomyopathy, which is potentially reversible – if recognized!

○   **What is the most common etiology of systolic heart failure and what EKG finding would make you suspicious of it?**

Coronary artery disease. Q waves on the EKG strongly suggest myocardial damage from this etiology.

...tionship between the serum sodium concentration and survival in systolic heart

...ed. The lower the serum sodium, the worse the prognosis.

...who carry the diagnosis of heart failure, what number have normal systolic

...licated diastolic dysfunction as a major factor in heart failure.

...man with anterior wall dyskinesis on echocardiogram and Q waves across the ..., was found during uncomplicated cardiac catheterization to have severe three ...ry disease, and a left ventricular end diastolic pressure of 30 mm Hg (BP 100/90). ...75 cc IV contrast and 50 cc/hour normal saline for 6 hours after the procedure. ...aluate him for acute dyspnea. Exam: BP is 150/80, HR is 140, RR is 30. JVD ...t. EKG: sinus tachycardia, IVCD, and 5 mm precordial ST elevations (baseline: ...). Should you administer thrombolysis for acute MI in the absence of chest pain?

...fluid gains and erroneous EKG interpretation in patients with reduced LV systolic ...nt had received almost half a liter of fluid. His LVEDP was very elevated – although ...onic and compensated elevation – and this additional fluid "tipped him over". His ...EKG suggest old MI and LV aneurysm: ST elevations can often worsen with ...situation. The patient improved rapidly with diuresis and IV nitroglycerin for blood ...cidentally, administration of thrombolytics in this patient post recent catheterization ...ead to severe bleeding from the puncture site.

...ld man with a history of intravenous drug use is receiving appropriate antibiotic ...rial endocarditis. Echocardiogram on presentation revealed vegetations on the ...no aortic regurgitation. You are called to his bedside to evaluate sudden onset of ...th. On exam, the patient is sitting bolt-upright in bed. He is dyspneic and ...is 140, BP is 110/80, heart exam reveals S1 faintly audible and the patient's rapid ...it difficult to appreciate murmurs. Rales throughout both lung fields, and ...s are normal. Given the paucity of findings are heard suggestive of aortic ...R), what is your working diagnosis?

...urgitation! Acute AR is notorious for its *lack* of findings that are typically seen in chronic ...idened pulse pressure, a prominent diastolic murmur and bounding peripheral pulses. ...ory, clues to the presence of AR include tachycardia and a soft S1.

...t should be emergently performed on this patient?

...ry edema in bacterial endocarditis warrants an immediate echocardiogram to evaluate the ...gies: mitral regurgitation and aortic insufficiency.

...ocardiography, what mitral valve finding is highly suggestive of acute, severe AI?

Premature closure of the mitral valve. High left ventricular diastolic pressures will cause the mitral valve leaflets to close early in diastole; this is the mechanism behind the soft first heart sound noted above on physical exam.

○ **Sustained ventricular tachycardia is well controlled in a 55 year-old man post non-Q wave MI with lidocaine 2 microgram/ml. He has a known history of ischemic cardiomyopathy. Day 3 of his admission, his speech becomes slurred, he is lethargic, and, when aroused, becomes very agitated. What should you do?**

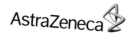

This patient has classic findings of lidocaine toxicity, and you should strongly consider stopping this drug. Elderly patients and patients with heart failure of hepatic insufficiency are especially at risk.

○   **What aspects of the history, physical exam, CXR, ECG and echocardiogram suggest systolic dysfunction and which suggest diastolic dysfunction?**

History	Systolic dysfunction	Diastolic dysfunction
Coronary artery disease	++++	+
Hypertension	++	++++
Diabetes Mellitus	+++	+
Valvular heart disease	++++	--
Paroxysmal dyspnea	++	+++

Physical Examination		
Cardiomegaly	+++	+
Soft heart sounds	++++	+
S3 gallop	+++	+
S4 gallop	+	+++
Hypertension	++	++++
Mitral regurgitation	+++	+
Aortic stenosis	+	++++
Rales	++	++
Edema	+++	+
Jugular venous distension	+++	+

Chest X-ray		
Cardiomegaly	+++	+
Pulmonary congestion	+++	+++

Electrocardiography		
Low voltage	+++	--
LVH	++	++++
LBBB	++++	++
Q waves	++	+

Echocardiography		
Low ejection fraction	++++	--
Left ventricular dilatation	++	--
LVH	++	++++

+ signs indicate "suggestive" (the number reflect the relative weight); -- signs indicate not very suggestive

○   **How can one differentiate between cardiogenic and noncardiogenic pulmonary edema based on the protein content of edema fluid?**

Noncardiogenic pulmonary edema has a edema protein to serum protein ratio of > 0.7 whereas in cardiogenic pulmonary edema, the edema protein to serum protein ratio is < 0.5.

○   **What are the functional and anatomical abnormalities associated with hypertrophic cardiomyopathy?**

- Diastolic dysfunction with impaired relaxation and distensibility
- Normal to increased left ventricular ejection fraction
- Narrowed left ventricular outflow tract with variable and labile LV outflow pressure gradient
- Frequent myocardial ischemia with frequent symptoms of angina and dyspnea
- Normal to decreased LV chamber size
- Systolic anterior motion of the anterior leaflet of the mitral valve in those cases with a LV outflow gradient
- Mitral regurgitation
- Increased diastolic filling pressures
- High percentage of ventricular and atrial arrhythmias
- Increased incidence of coronary artery disease in patients over age 45
- Poor predictability of electrophysiology studies and ambulatory ECG monitoring for assessing risk of sudden death
- Pulmonary hypertension in 25% of cases
- Impaired vasodilatory reserve
- Significantly increased myocardial oxygen demand due to increased wall stress.

○ What is the hallmark of treatment for hypertrophic cardiomyopathy?

Beta-blockers. They are the most useful and most efficacious agents. Calcium channel blockers, most notably verapamil, are a reasonable alternative in patients with contraindications or intolerability to beta-blockers, but nifedipine and diltiazem are considerably less efficacious then verapamil. DDD pacing is helpful about 10% of cases and septal myomectomy is very helpful in patients with LV outflow gradients above 50 mm Hg or in those who do not respond satisfactorily to medical therapy.

○ What disease does restrictive cardiomyopathies resemble from a functional standpoint?

Constrictive pericarditis.

○ What is the hallmark of restrictive cardiomyopathy?

Abnormal diastolic function with impaired ventricular filling from rigid ventricular walls. Systolic function is often unimpaired.

○ What is the characteristic feature of restrictive cardiomyopathy?

Like constrictive pericarditis, it is a deep and rapid early decline in ventricular pressure at the onset of diastole with a rapid rise to a plateau in early diastole.

○ What are the hemodynamic features seen on cardiac catheterization in restrictive cardiomyopathy?

- Prominent y descent followed by a rapid rise and plateau on atrial pressure tracing
- Frequent rapid x descent. When this is present, along with the prominent y descent and rise, this results in the characteristic M or W waveform in the atrial pressure tracing.
- Characteristic "square root" sign consisting in a deep and rapid early decline in ventricular pressure at the onset of diastole with a rapid rise to a plateau in early diastole.
- Elevated systemic and pulmonary venous pressures with elevated pulmonary artery pressures (usually greater than 50 mm Hg).
- LV filling pressures higher than RV filling pressures by more than 5 mm Hg (distinguishes from constrictive pericarditis where the difference is less than 5 mm Hg).

○ What percentage of cases can the distinction between restrictive cardiomyopathy and constrictive pericarditis **not** be made on hemodynamic grounds?

25%.

○ What is the most frequent symptom reported in restrictive cardiomyopathy?

Exercise intolerance with dyspnea on exertion.

O   **What is the prognosis of restrictive cardiomyopathy?**

Highly variable but usually one of relentless symptomatic progression and high mortality. No specific therapy is available (except in cases due to iron overload), although calcium antagonists may be of some value.

O   **What are the clinical features of cardiac amyloidosis?**

*   CHF, predominantly right sided with peripheral edema and JVD
*   Less commonly is left-sided CHF due to systolic dysfunction (this manifestation responds poorly to treatment and has a very poor prognosis).
*   Orthostatic hypotension, occuring in about 10% of cases.
*   Conduction system abnormalities with arrhythmias, least common mode of presentation. Sudden cardiac death, in this subset, is high.

O   **Which medications have to be used very cautiously in patients with cardiac amyloidosis?**

Digoxin and nifedipine. Digoxin can cause serious arrhythmias in these patients and nifedipine can worsen CHF due to its binding to amyloid fibrils.

O   **What is the treatment and prognosis of cardiac amyloidosis?**

The prognosis is generally poor and the treatment is supportive only, with diuretics and vasodilators being the mainstays.

O   **What are the common cardiac clinical manifestations of sarcoidosis?**

Sudden death is common, due to the high incidence of ventricular arrhythmias, especially VT. Conduction system abnormalities, particularly high degree AV block, are common, due to the affinity of sarcoidosis for the AV node and His bundle. Congestive heart failure, predominantly right-sided, is common and pericardial effusions occur in about 20% of cases.

ELECTROCARDIOGRAPHY AND CARDIAC ELECTROPHYSIOLOGY

○ **What are the most common causes of MAT (multifocal atrial tachycardia)?**

COPD with exacerbation is the most common cause, followed by CHF, sepsis and methylxanthine toxicity. Treatment consists of treatment of the underlying disorder as well as the use of verapamil, magnesium, or digoxin for slowing the arrythmia.

○ **How is atrial flutter treated?**

Initiate A-V nodal blockade with beta-adrenergic blocking agents, calcium channel blockers or digoxin to slow the rate. Once this is accomplished, treat a stable patient with chemical cardioversion using a class 1A agent, such as quinidine or procainamide. If this fails to convert the patient, or the patient is unstable, synchronized electrocardioversion should be attempted starting at 25-50 Joules.

○ **What are the most common causes of atrial fibrillation?**

Hypertension with hypertensive heart disease is very common. Ischemic heart disease, mitral or aortic valvular heart disease, cor pulmonale, dilated cardiomyopathy, hypertrophic cardiomyopathy (particularly the obstructive type), alcohol intoxication ("holiday heart syndrome"), hypo- or hyperthyroidism, pulmonary embolism, sepsis, hypoxia, pre-excitation syndrome and pericarditis are also common causes.

○ **How is atrial fibrillation treated?**

The treatment of atrial fibrillation consists of three major considerations: 1) control of ventricular rate, 2) conversion, if possible or feasible, to sinus rhythm, and 3) prevention of thromboembolic events, particularly CVA. Rate control is best managed with beta-adrenergic blockers or calcium channel blockers (diltiazem or verapamil), or less desirable, digoxin. Digoxin should be used in patients with poor LV systolic function and those with a contraindication to beta-blockers and calcium channel blockers. Digoxin provides good rate control at rest but often suboptimal rate control during exertion. Conversion to sinus rhythm, in the stable patient, is best managed, initially, with antiarrhythmic agents, such as 1A agents like quinidine or procainamide, 1C agents such as propafenone or Class III agents like amiodarone or sotalol. In the unstable patient or the patient with acute ischemia, hypotension or pulmonary edema, immediate synchronized electrical cardioversion, starting at 200 joules should be performed. If, in the stable patient, cardioversion with antiarrhythmic agents is unsuccessful, synchronized electrical cardioversion should be performed without interruption of antiarrhythmic therapy. Patients with atrial fibrillation of 1 year duration or longer, or those with left atrial size of >5.0 cm on echocardiography should not be cardioverted because of the extremely low success rate. Patients with recent atrial fibrillation >3 days duration should be started on Warfarin and anticoagulated to an INR between 2-3.5 for at least three weeks before any attempt to cardiovert to sinus rhythm because of the significant risk of embolic CVA. Those patients with chronic atrial fibrillation should be on lifelong Warfarin, unless an absolute contraindication to Warfarin exists or the patient cannot reliably take Warfarin.

○ **What percentage of patients with atrial fibrillation converted to sinus rhythm will revert back into atrial fibrillation?**

50% will revert back to atrial fibrillation within one year of cardioversion, regardless of medical therapy.

O   **What is the risk of CVA in patients with atrial fibrillation with and without anticoagulation?**

Patients with atrial fibrillation not anticoagulated with warfarin have a 25% incidence of CVA within 5 years (5% per year). Those patients anticoagulated to therapeutic levels have a 4% incidence of CVA within 5 years (0.8% per year) Aspirin is a clearly inferior substitute to warfarin, but is much preferable to no anticoagulant or antithrombotic therapy.

O   **What is the most common mechanism responsible for supraventricular tachycardia (SVT)?**

A-V node reentry.

O   **What arrhythmia is likely in a 20 year-old man presenting with lightheadedness, and a wide-complex, irregular tachycardia of 220 beats per minute and QRS complexes of varying morphology?**

Atrial fibrillation conducting rapidly down an accessory pathway (in WPW).

O   **What are the common causes of SVT?**

Myocardial ischemia, myocardial infarction, congestive heart failure, pericarditis, rheumatic heart disease, mitral valve prolapse, pre-excitation syndromes, COPD, ethanol intoxication, hypoxia, pneumonia, sepsis and digoxin toxicity.

O   **What is the treatment of paroxysmal SVT?**

In a hemodynamically stable patient, intravenous adenosine. If unsuccessful, then intravenous verapamil, beta-blockers or procainamide. In the unstable patient with hypotension, angina, or heart failure, immediate synchronized cardioversion should be performed.

O   **What is the most common supraventricular arrhythmia in the perioperative setting?**

Atrial fibrillation.

O   **You are called to the Cardiothoracic ICU to evaluate the sudden onset of hypotension in an 80 year-old woman. She received a porcine aortic valve for severe aortic stenosis less than 24 hours ago. The bedside monitor reveals atrial fibrillation at a rate of 120 bpm. What is the pathophysiology?**

A rapid ventricular response and loss of AV synchrony, as can be seen in new-onset atrial fibrillation, can have devastating hemodynamic consequences, especially in patients with impaired diastolic filling – often including the elderly, and patients with left ventricular hypertrophy, which this patient with long-standing aortic stenosis most likely has.

O   **What pharmacotherapy is most appropriate in the above patient?**

None. Hemodynamically unstable patients with tachyarrhythmias are best treated with electrical cardioversion.

O   **What is the key feature of Mobitz Type I 2° AV block (Wenckebach)?**

A progressive prolongation of the PR interval until the atrial impulse is no longer conducted through to the ventricle, resulting in a dropped QRS. Almost always transient, atropine and transcutaneous/transvenous pacing is required for the rare instances of symptoms or cardiac instability.

O   **What is the feature of Mobitz II 2° AV block?**

A constant PR interval until one sinus beat fails to conduct through to the ventricle, resulting in a dropped QRS. Since this rhythm is indicative of His bundle damage, and 85% of patients with this rhythm eventually develop complete heart block, temporary followed by permanent pacing is usually required.

○ **What is the most common cause of Mobitz Type II 2° AV block?**

Coronary artery disease with acute myocardial ischemia. In the absence of coronary artery disease, the most common cause is degenerative AV node and His bundle disease.

○ **What is the appropriate management of the above arrhythmia in a patient on no SA or AV nodal suppressant drugs?**

Temporary transvenous pacemaker insertion followed by permanent pacemaker implantation.

○ **A 57 year-old male is scheduled for a total colectomy for ulcerative colitis. He has stable angina for several years and has hypertension. His pre-op ECG reveals NSR, LVH and 1° AV block. What is the likelihood of high degree AV block occurring in the perioperative period?**

Patients with 1° AV block have an extremely low incidence of developing high degree AV block in the perioperative period or any other period. Thus, no temporary pacing in the perioperative period is required.

○ **A 26 year-old male present to your clinic for an insurance physical. An ECG reveals Wolff-Parkinson-White syndrome. He is asymptomatic and has no history of palpitations or arrhythmia. What is the most appropriate management of this patient?**

No therapy or work-up is required at this time since there is no evidence that the risk of sudden death can be safely mitigated or that individuals with asymptomatic WPW can be reliably risk stratified with regard to sudden death.

○ **What is the most commonly occurring form of ventricular tachycardia?**

Ventricular tachycardia (VT) occurring in patients with healed myocardial infarction. Other causes include bundle branch reentry VT, VT of right ventricular outflow tract origin, idiopathic left ventricular tachycardia, drug-induced VT (proarrhythmia), and VT due to right ventricular dysplasia. Rare causes include long QT syndrome and lymphocytic myocarditis.

○ **A 48 year-old male with no history of angina, MI or other cardiac symptoms is referred to you for evaluation of palpitations. A 24-hour Holter monitor reveals four three-beat runs of ventricular tachycardia without any symptoms. The patient has no risk factors for coronary artery disease, is a non-smoker, and has a normal resting ECG. His echocardiogram is normal. What is the best management strategy for this patient?**

No therapy or further work-up is required. The patient should be reassured that the risk of sudden death is very low and that medical therapy will either worsen his arrhythmia or be of no significant benefit.

○ **A 28 year-old male with two previous episodes of palpitations and shortness of breath in the last year is brought in to the Emergency Department by paramedics with severe palpitations, hypotension and shortness of breath. His BP is 90/55 and his HR is 195/minute. A rhythm strip reveals narrow complex QRS tachycardia. A 12-lead ECG reveals what appears to be atrial fibrillation. Synchronized cardioversion is successful in terminating the arrhythmia, and the post-cardioversion ECG reveals Wolff-Parkinson-White syndrome. What is the most appropriate management strategy in this patient?**

Electrophysiology testing with intracardiac mapping, followed by catheter ablation of the accessory conduction pathway.

○   A 67 year-old woman with severe 3-vessel coronary artery disease with very small distal vessels, deemed inoperable, is brought into the Emergency Department following a syncopal episode. The paramedics caught the final beats of what looked like a wide-complex QRS tachycardia on a rhythm strip and you confirm this on inspection of the tracing. She is now awake, alert and breathing comfortably. An echocardiogram performed one month ago revealed a dilated left ventricle with poor systolic function (estimated ejection fraction ~ 20-25%). What is the most appropriate management strategy for this patient?

Empiric therapy with Amiodarone.

○   What percentage of patients treated with long-term Amiodarone for ventricular tachycardia will develop bradycardia that requires permanent pacing?

15%.

○   What percentage of patients who undergo CABG develop post-operative atrial fibrillation?

33%.

○   What are the most common independent risk factors for the development of post-operative atrial fibrillation following CABG?

Right coronary artery disease with bypass grafting of the RCA, hypertension, prior myocardial infarction, history of paroxysmal atrial fibrillation and decreased LV systolic function.

○   What is the preferred management strategy of immediate post-operative atrial fibrillation in patients following CABG?

Unless contraindicated, beta-blockers are the preferred agent of choice, initially intravenous, then oral. When beta-blockers are contraindicated, calcium channel blockers, such as verapamil or diltiazem, are useful in slowing the ventricular rate, but they are not very effective in converting the rhythm back to sinus. Anti-arrhythmic agents, such as propafenone, flecainide or the IA class of quinidine/procainamide are useful in converting the rhythm to sinus. The majority of patients who develop post-op atrial fibrillation will spontaneously convert to sinus rhythm or can be converted with the above agents. Those who remain in atrial fibrillation for more than 48 hours must be started on full anticoagulation with heparin followed by coumadin, as the risk of stroke is quite high. Those patients who remain in atrial fibrillation for more than 1 week post-operatively have a high incidence of recurrent atrial fibrillation following cardioversion and will likely revert to chronic atrial fibrillation within 1-3 months after surgery. Those patients with low ejection fractions can have their arrhythmia well-managed with digoxin.

○   What is the most common cause of multifocal atrial tachycardia?

Chronic obstructive or restrictive lung disease with acute exacerbation, often with cor pulmonale. Other causes include CHF, pulmonary embolism, coronary artery disease and severe mitral stenosis.

○   What is the most effective treatment of multifocal atrial tachycardia?

Treat the underlying cause. In most cases, that begins with treating the acute exacerbation of lung disease and reducing the resultant pulmonary hypertension and hypoxemia that exists. The arrhythmia is best managed by trying to slow the ventricular rate with calcium channel blockers, such as verapamil or diltiazem, or less favorably with digoxin.

○   What is the most common electrophysiologic cause of supraventricular tachycardia?

AV node reentry.

○ **What type of supraventricular tachycardias are due to ectopic atrial phenomenon?**

Multifocal atrial tachycardia and ectopic junctional tachycardia.

○ **How does one differentiate a reentry supraventricular tachycardia from an ectopic supraventricular tachycardia?**

Automatic ectopic SVT's exhibit the following features: 1) the presence of a "warm-up" (progressive acceleration for the first few beats), 2) sameness of all the ectopic P waves in the tachycardia, including the first ectopic beat of the tachycardia, and 3) a premature stimulus resetting the tachycardia (similar to the way a PAC resets the sinus rhythm). Reentry SVT's lack a "warm-up and a premature stimulus does not reset the arrhythmia, but in fact, may terminate the tachycardia. Reentry SVT's also exhibit prolongation of the first ectopic P-R interval and the initial ectopic P wave differs from the subsequent ectopic retrograde P waves of the tachycardia. Additional clues that favor a reentry tachycardia include the presence of ventricular aberration, initiation of the tachycardia when the sinus rate accelerates without the presence of a PAC or prolongation of the P-R interval, incessant form of the tachycardia, and the association of retrograde ectopic P waves with an R-P' interval shorter than the P-R.

○ **What are the salient features of SVT?**

1. Rapid (rate between 100-250/min), regular, normal QRS complexes.
2. Abnormal P waves constantly related to QRS (may not be discernible).
3. ST-T depression frequently seen.

○ **What is the earliest ECG finding in hyperkalemia?**

Tall, symmetrically peaked T waves.

○ **What are the ECG criteria of cor pulmonale without obstructive airway disease?**

1. Right-axis deviation with a mean QRS axis to the right of + 110°.
2. R/S amplitude ratio in V1 > 1.
3. R/S amplitude ratio in V6 < 1.
4. Clockwise rotation of the electrical axis.
5. S1-Q3 or S1-S2-S3 pattern.
6. Normal voltage QRS.

○ **What are the ECG criteria of cor pulmonale with obstructive airway disease?**

1. Isoelectric P waves in lead I or right-axis deviation of the P vector.
2. P-pulmonale pattern (an increase in P-wave amplitude in II, III, aVF).
3. Tendency for right-axis deviation of the QRS.
4. R/S amplitude ratio in V6 <1.
5. Low-voltage QRS.
6. S1-Q3 or S1-S2-S3 pattern.
7. Incomplete RBBB.
8. R/S amplitude ratio in V1 > 1.
9. Marked clockwise rotation of the electrical axis.
10. Occasional large Q wave or QS in the inferior or mid-precordial leads, suggesting healed myocardial infarction.

○ **What are the electrocardiographic findings in pulmonary embolism?**

1. Incomplete or complete RBBB.
2. S in lead I and aVL > 1.5 mm.

3. Transition zone shift to V5 (late transition).
4. QS in leads III and aVF, but not in lead II.
5. QRS axis > 90° or indeterminate axis.
6. Low limb lead voltage
7. T wave inversion in leads III and aVF or in leads V1-V4.

○ What is the electrocardiographic hallmark of hypothermia?

Osborne waves, the characteristic deflection of the terminal portion of the QRS. Sinus bradycardia is usually present, and atrial fibrillation and conduction system disturbances can occur.

○ What is the electrocardiographic criteria for LVH?

Scott's criteria for LVH consists of the following:
1. R wave in lead I and S wave in lead III more than 25 mm.
2. R wave in aVL more than 7.5 mm.
3. R wave in aVF more than 20 mm.
4. S wave in aVR more than 14 mm.
5. S wave in V1 or V2 + R wave in V5 or V6 more than 35 mm.
6. R wave in V5 or V6 more than 26 mm.
7. R wave + S wave in any V lead more than 45 mm.

○ What is the significance of ST-T abnormalities associated with LVH?

It is a marker for the presence of coronary artery disease and a risk factor for increased cardiac morbidity and mortality.

○ What is the ECG criteria for RVH?

1. Reversal of precordial pattern with tall R wave over right precordium (V1,V2) and deep S wave over left precordium (V5,V6), or rS over entire precordium.
2. Normal QRS interval.
3. Late intrinsicoid deflection in V1-V2.
4. Right axis deviation.
5. ST segment depression with upward convexity and inverted T waves in right precordial leads (V1-V2) and in whichever limb leads show tall R waves.

○ What are the salient features of LBBB?

1. QS or rS in lead V1.
2. Late intrinsicoid deflection without Q waves and monophasic R wave in lead V6.
3. Monophasic R wave and no Q waves in lead I.
4. QRS interval greater than .12 seconds.
5. Normal QRS axis.
6. ST-T wave repolarization abnormalities with T wave axis opposite of QRS axis in all precordial leads and in leads I and aVL.

○ What are the salient features of RBBB?

1. Late intrinsicoid deflection with M-shaped QRS (RSR' variant) or qR in lead V1.
2. Early intrinsicoid deflection and wide, deep S wave in lead V6.
3. Wide S wave in lead I.
4. QRS interval > .12 seconds.
5. Normal QRS axis.
6. ST-T wave repolarization abnormalities with T wave opposite of QRS axis in leads V1-V2.

○   **What is the criteria for left anterior hemiblock?**

1. Left axis deviation (usually > -35°).
2. Small Q in lead I and aVL, small R in lead II,III, and aVF.
3. Normal QRS duration, although QRS interval usually between .09 and .12 seconds.
4. Late intrinsicoid deflection in aVL.
5. Increased QRS voltage in limb leads.
6. Terminal R wave peak in lead aVR later than terminal R wave peak in lead aVL.

○   **What are the criteria for left posterior hemiblock?**

1. Right axis deviation (usually > +120°).
2. Small R wave in lead I and aVL, and small Q wave in leads II,III, and aVF.
3. Normal QRS duration.
4. Late intrinsicoid deflection in lead aVF.
5. No evidence for RVH.
6. Terminal R wave peak in lead aVR earlier than terminal R wave peak in lead aVL.

○   **Can RBBB be found in patients with no structural heart disease? LBBB?**

RBBB can frequently be found in patients without structural heart disease, although in older patients, it frequently occurs in the setting of CAD, valvular heart disease or cardiomyopathy. LBBB, on the other hand, almost always occurs in the setting of structural heart disease and rarely is found in healthy patients. LBBB usually occurs in patients with LV systolic dysfunction, with or without coronary artery disease.

○   **What are the indications for intracardiac electrophysiologic study of sinus node function?**

1. To assess symptomatic patients in whom sinus node dysfunction is suspected to the cause of symptoms, but a causal relation between an arrhythmia and the symptoms has not been established after appropriate evaluation with 24-hour ambulatory monitoring, exercise stress testing or prolonged inpatient cardiac monitoring.
2. To assess patients who have documented sinus node dysfunction in whom evaluation of AV or VA conduction or susceptibility to arrhythmias may aid in the selection of the most appropriate modality.
3. To assess patients with electrocardiographically documented sinus bradyarrhythmias to determine if abnormalities are due to intrinsic disease, autonomic nervous system dysfunction, or the effects of drugs to help select therapeutic options.

○   **What are the indications for intracardiac electrophysiologic study of patients with unexplained syncope?**

1. In patients with syncope that remains unexplained after appropriate evaluation, and who have suspected structural heart disease.
2. In patients with recurrent unexplained syncope without structural heart disease and a negative head-up tilt test.

○   **What are the indications for intracardiac electrophysiologic study of patients with wide-complex tachycardias?**

In patients with wide QRS tachycardias when the correct diagnosis in unclear after analysis of available ECG tracings and knowledge of the correct diagnosis is necessary for appropriate patient care.

○   **What are the indications for intracardiac electrophysiologic study of patients with narrow QRS tachycardia?**

1. In patients with frequent of poorly tolerated episodes of tachcardia not adequately responding to drug therapy in whom information about site of origin, mechanism, and electrophysiological properties of

the tachycardia pathways is essential for choosing appropriate therapy (drugs, catheter ablation, pacing, or surgery).

2.   In patients who prefer ablative therapy to drug therapy.
3.   In patients with frequent episodes of tachycardia requiring drug treatment in whom there is concern about proarrhythmia or the effects of antiarrhythmic drug therapy on sinus node or AV node conduction.

O   What are the indications for intracardiac electrophysiologic study in patients who are survivors of cardiac arrest?

1.   In patients surviving an episode of cardiac arrest without evidence of an acute Q-wave myocardial infarction.
2.   In patients surviving an episode of cardiac arrest occurring > 48 hours after acute myocardial infarction.
3.   In patients surviving cardiac arrest due to bradyarrhythmias.
4.   In patients surviving cardiac arrest thought to be associated with a congenital repolarization abnormality (e.g., long Q-T syndrome) in whom the results of noninvasive diagnostic testing are equivocal.

O   What are the indications for intracardiac electrophysiologic study in patients with acquired AV block?

1.   In symptomatic patients where suspected His-Purkinje block has not been established as a cause of symptoms.
2.   In patients with 2° or 3° AV block treated with a pacemaker remain symptomatic where another arrhythmia is suspected to be the cause of symptoms.
3.   In patients with 2° or 3° AV block where knowledge of the site of block or its mechanism, or response to drug therapy or other temporary intervention may help to direct therapy or assess prognosis.
4.   In patients with premature concealed junctional depolarizations suspected as a cause of 2° or 3° AV block.

O   Which patients are programmed electrical stimulation (PES) indicated for to determine guidance of drug therapy?

1.   Those patients with sustained ventricular tachycardia (VT) or cardiac arrest, especially those with prior myocardial infarction.
2.   Those patients with AV node reentrant tachycardia, AV reentrant tachycardia using an accessory pathway or atrial fibrillation associated with an accessory pathway in whom drug therapy is involved.
3.   Those patients with sinus node reentrant tachycardia, atrial tachycardia, atrial fibrillation or atrial flutter without ventricular preexcitation syndrome in whom chronic drug therapy is planned.
4.   Those patients with arrhythmias not inducible during controlled electrophysiologic study in whom drug therapy is planned.

O   What is the most common form of AV reentry?

Orthodromic reentry in the WPW syndrome (Wolff-Parkinson-White).

O   What is the significance of ST depression during SVT?

It is a benign condition and is related to repolarization abnormalities from reentry rather than ischemia.

O   Can one reliably identify high-risk asymptomatic patients for medical or surgical therapy in patients with ventricular preexcitation by measuring the effective refractory period of the accessory pathway?

No. They are nonspecific and are not predictive of high risk, even in symptomatic patients.

O   **What is the agent of choice for the immediate pharmacologic conversion of atrial fibrillation to sinus rhythm of less than 48 hours duration?**

Ibutilide.

O   **What is the treatment of Torsades de Pointes?**

Torsades de Pointes is a polymorphic form of ventricular tachycardia that occurs in the setting of long repolarization. Treatment usually requires removal of the reversible triggers that caused Q-T prolongation, such as hypokalemia and drugs, such as quinidine and other antiarrhythmic agents, pacing the atrium or ventricle to increase cardiac rate and rapidly infusing magnesium sulfate.

O   **What is the treatment of hereditary prolonged Q-T syndrome?**

Beta-blockers, cervicothoracic sympathomimectomy, chronic pacing and the implantable cardioverter/defibrillator.

O   **What is the most common form of ventricular tachycardia?**

VT due to healed myocardial infarction.

O   **What are the classes of sustained, monomorphic VT?**

1.   VT due to healed myocardial infarction
2.   Bundle branch reentry VT
3.   VT of right ventricular outflow tract origin
4.   Idiopathic left VT
5.   Drug-induced VT
6.   VT due to right ventricular dysplasia

O   **Which classes of sustained, monomorphic VT can occur in the absence of structural heart disease?**

VT of right ventricular outflow tract origin and idiopathic left VT. Both occur in young people with normal hearts. Exercise-induced VT is typically of right ventricular outflow tract origin.

O   **What types of VT are catheter ablation effective in treating?**

Bundle-branch reentry VT, right ventricular outflow tract VT, and idiopathic VT.

O   **How common is bundle branch reentry VT?**

6% of all VT.

O   **What is the mechanism of bundle branch reentry VT?**

The circuit of reentry is thought to consist of the right and left bundle branches and intervening myocardium. Reentry may proceed in either direction, and virtually all patients with this type of VT have His-Purkinje disease, with resultant HV interval prolongation and intraventricular conduction delay. However, they do not have complete bundle branch block. This arrhythmia has a predilection for idiopathic dilated cardiomyopathy.

O   **What features should make you suspect VT of right ventricular outflow tract origin?**

Occurrence in young people with otherwise no structural heart disease when a left bundle branch morphology of VT is observed. This form is often exercise-induced. Anti-adrenergic therapy is often effective as is catheter ablation.

O   **What features should make you suspect VT of idiopathic left ventricular type?**

Also occurring in young people, the ECG typically shows RBBB and left axis deviation. Verapamil or catheter ablation are the most effective therapies.

O   **What is right ventricular dysplasia?**

A rare myocardial disease that causes fibrosis and fatty replacement of the right ventricle primarily. Sustained VT, both monomorphic and polymorphic, is a common manifestation of the disease and a genetic abnormality is responsible for the disease.

O   **What is lymphocytic myocarditis?**

A form of myocarditis that may commonly present with VT or sudden death as its initial manifestation. In some cases, ventricular dysfunction is minimal or absent. This entity is difficult to diagnose and therapeutic decisions are complex.

O   **In a patient with a wide-complex QRS tachycardia who is hemodynamically stable, what is the agent of choice as initial treatment?**

Lidocaine. The treatment of wide-complex QRS tachycardias that prove to be VT, rather than SVT, with verapamil have resulted in hypotension and cardiac arrest. Adenosine is an alternative that is gaining favor in that its half-life is very short (10 seconds) and it carries no long-term risk of cardiac deterioration. The rule of thumb is to treat all wide-complex QRS tachycardias as VT until proven otherwise, and administer lidocaine.

O   **What is the significance of a positive head-up tilt test in a patient with syncope?**

Most patients with syncope with positive tilt tests have vasodepressor syncope (common faint).

O   **What are common causes for tachyarrhythmias in the ICU patient?**

At baseline, ICU patients are "stressed out", have fluids and drugs pumped in and out of them. Always consider catecholamines, cardiac ischemia, drug toxicity (iatrogenic or otherwise) and electrolyte imbalance (i.e., hypokalemia) as etiologies for arrhythmias, tachy or otherwise.

O   **You note sinus tachycardia, low voltage, and alternating QRS voltages with every beat in a hypotensive patient with renal failure. What is your diagnosis?**

EKG findings of sinus tachycardia, low QRS voltage and electrical alternans in a patient with renal failure all point to cardiac tamponade as the cause of hypotension.

O   **What are effective treatments for vasodepressor syncope (vasovagal syncope)?**

Beta-blockers or disopyramide, to reduce left ventricular inotropy and vagal tone. Support stockings are useful in reducing peripheral blood pooling. Scopolamine can be useful in preventing bradycardia and blunt the peripheral arterial dilatation. Theophylline has had some success as well.

O   **What is the prognosis of patients with syncope of unknown etiology?**

Those with syncope unexplained after neurologic, electrophysiologic and tilt testing have a fairly good prognosis, though not that of a normal population. Those with structural heart disease are at greater risk for sudden death, while those without cardiac disease are at minimal risk of premature death.

○ **What is the normal response to head-up tilting?**

An increase in heart rate with minimal change in mean arterial blood pressure.

○ **What types of abnormal responses to head-up tilting are there?**

The first is a cardioinhibitory response, consisting of bradycardia usually in association with a fall in blood pressure. The second response is a pure vasodepressor reaction in which the blood pressure falls with an increase or slight decrease in heart rate.

○ **What is the significance of reduced heart rate variability?**

This often occurs in congestive heart failure. Reduced heart rate variability has been found to be a strong predictor of subsequent mortality in a postinfarction population, regardless of left ventricular function.

○ **What are the criteria for the identification of late potentials on the Signal-Averaged electrocardiogram?**

No intraventricular conduction delay on ECG
1. LAS40 > 38 ms, or
2. RMS40 < 20 microvolts

Left Bundle Branch Block
1. LAS40 > 55 ms, and
2. RMS40 < 17 microvolts

There is no specific established criteria in the presence of RBBB and non-specific IVCD.

○ **What specific circumstances is there general agreement that antiarrhythmic therapy is not indicated?**

1. Asymptomatic atrial ectopy and unsustained SVT.
2. Asymptomatic ventricular ectopy without runs of VT.
3. Simple ventricular ectopy in the setting of acute myocardial infarction. Due to recent evidence that lidocaine may cause sinus arrest, AV block, and other adverse effects that outweigh its potential to prevent VF, it should not be used except when ectopy is so frequent and so timed that it significantly impairs hemodynamics.
4. Asymptomatic, unsustained VT in the absence of structural heart disease or other risk factors.
5. Asymptomatic patients with WPW syndrome (without known SVT). There is no evidence that the risk of sudden death can safely be mitigated or that individuals at risk can be identified in this population.
6. Mildly symptomatic patients with simple ventricular or atrial ectopy. Reassurance of these patients, rather than drug therapy is preferred.

○ **Name five useful ECG criteria for identifying VT.**

1. AV dissociation – often best seen in lead V1 and rare in SVT with aberrancy.
2. Capture of fusion beats – often noted as a "narrow" premature beat occurring during a wide complex tachycardia.
3. A QRS with a RBBB morphology greater than 140ms in duration, or a LBBB morphology greater than 160ms in duration.
4. Extreme right or left axis deviation ("northwest axis") is seldom seen outside of Vt.
5. Positive or negative concordance of QRS complexes in the precordial leads.

O   **Which antiarrhythmic agents increase defibrillation threshold (i.e., increase the energy requirement for successful defibrillation)?**

Lidocaine, mexiletine, encainide, flecainide, propafenone, amiodarone and verapamil.

O   **Which agents decrease defibrillation threshold?**

Sotalol, and amiodarone in the presence of acute myocardial ischemia.

O   **What are some of the arrhythmias treated by catheter ablation and what are the success rates?**

1) WPW accessory pathway syndrome	95%
2) AV block with rapid ventricular response	90%
3) AV node reentry	90%
4) RV outflow tract VT	90%
5) Bundle branch reentry VT	95%
6) RV dysplasia VT	60%
7) VT due to healed myocardial infarction	30%
8) Ectopic atrial tachycardia	90%

O   **A 73 year-old patient with coronary artery disease and an old anterior wall myocardial infarction is on digoxin therapy and is referred to you for evaluation of recurrent episodes of VT. During PES, the tachycardia can be initiated by rapid pacing, but it cannot be initiated or terminated by single premature stimuli. Rapid pacing accelerates the rate of the tachycardia. What is the most likely mechanism for this arrhythmia?**

Triggered automaticity.

O   **Late potentials have been shown to give prognostic information concerning the risk of sudden cardiac death in which patients?**

Patients with recent myocardial infarction.

O   **What is the appropriate management of incessant VT caused by IC antiarrhythmic agents, such as flecainide?**

Discontinuation of the agent, bed rest, correction of acidosis and pharmacologic support of hypotension. Temporary pacing is of no value in proarrhythmia, but is effective in Torsades de Pointes caused by IA antiarrhythmic agents.

O   **What is pacemaker syndrome?**

Pacemaker syndrome is caused by pacing the ventricle asynchronously, so that VA conduction or AV dissociation occurs. Though hypotension is a common cause of symptoms during pacing, and manifests as weakness, other symptoms such as chest pain, shortness of breath and palpitations may occur without any decline in blood pressure. It does not seem to occur more commonly in heart failure. Converting patients to DDD pacing from VVI corrects the problem in most cases.

O   **What pacing mode is most appropriate for a 17 year-old woman with complete heart block following surgical repair of a small membranous VSD?**

DDD. Rate-responsive dual chamber pacing is unnecessary because sinus node function is expected to be normal.

○ **A 74 year-old, insulin-dependent diabetic male with severe triple-vessel CAD with small distal vessels, generalized poor left ventricular function (LVEF of 24%), and LBBB on ECG has recurrent VT with syncope. He has COPD with a maximum baseline pO2 of 48. He fails to respond to procainamide, mexiletine and the combination of the two. What is the best treatment alternative?**

Implantable defibrillator.

○ **What is the more common form of AV nodal reentry, orthodromic (slow-fast) or antidromic (fast-slow)?**

Orthodromic (slow-fast). It is usually triggered by an atrial premature beat associated with a prolonged P'-R interval. In these cases, the P' wave is often invisible in the surface ECG. Antidromic AV nodal reentry is more common in children.

○ **What are the most common initial rhythm in adults with cardiac arrest?**

VF and VT.

○ **For VF or unstable VT, what is the most important intervention to optimize chances for successful resuscitation?**

Defibrillation.

○ **What percentage of individuals successfully resuscitated from sudden cardiac death will succumb to a second episode within 2 years?**

60%.

○ **What is the primary indication for atropine?**

Symptomatic bradycardia.

○ **The most important action of epinephrine when used during resuscitation is?**

Alpha-adrenergic effect = vasoconstriction.

○ **What are the indications for calcium therapy?**

Documented or suspected hypocalcemia, hyperkalemia, hypermagnesemia, and calcium channel blocker overdose.

○ **What is the treatment of choice for patients with supraventricular tachycardia and cardiovascular compromise?**

Adenosine, but in the event that vascular access is not available quickly, synchronized cardioversion becomes the treatment of choice.

○ **When should atropine be used for the treatment of bradycardia?**

Only after adequate ventilation and oxygenation have been established, since hypoxemia is a common cause of bradycardia.

○ **T/F: Defibrillation is indicated for the treatment of asystole.**

False. Defibrillation is the definitive treatment for ventricular fibrillation or pulseless ventricular tachycardia. The treatment for asystole is epinephrine.

O   **After a cardiac arrest, what is the most common reason for poor perfusion?**

Cardiogenic shock resulting from arrest-associated myocardial ischemia.

O   **What are the only two pharmacologic agents that have been proven to improve survival in cardiac arrest?**

Epinephrine and atropine.

O   **Of all of the components of cardiopulmonary resuscitation as outlined by ACLS protocol, which has the greatest impact on survival?**

Adequacy of chest compression to maintain sufficient coronary perfusion pressure to sustain myocardial viability.

O   **What is the immediate treatment of choice in ventricular fibrillation?**

Immediate defibrillation, starting at 200 Joules. If unsuccessful, repeat at 300 Joules, and if still unsuccessful, repeat a third time at 360 Joules. If still unsuccessful, start CPR and achieve adequate ventilation with immediate intubation.

O   **What is the treatment of choice for hemodynamically stable ventricular tachycardia?**

Intravenous bolus of lidocaine at 1 mg/kg, followed by an infusion of lidocaine at 2-4 mg/min. A repeat bolus should be given at .5 mg/kg, 15 minutes after the initial bolus.

O   **In CPR, what is the ventilation to compression ratio for one rescuer? For two rescuers?**

1 rescuer: 2 breaths to 15 compressions
2 rescuers: 1 breath to 5 compressions

O   **Non-traumatic cardiac arrest patients are most likely to be successfully resuscitated from what abnormal rhythm?**

Ventricular fibrillation. Success is time dependent, generally declining at a rate of 2-10% per minute.

O   **How many deaths per year in the U.S. are due to cardiovascular disease?**

930,000, 43% of all deaths per year. More than 1/2 of all deaths occur in women. 2/3 of sudden deaths, due to CAD, take place outside the hospital, and most occur within 2 hours of the onset of symptoms.

O   **In a patient with ventricular fibrillation, what regimen should be used in the administration of bretylium?**

5 mg/kg IV bolus followed by 10 mg/kg IV bolus. The maximum dose is 30-35 mg/kg.

O   **What drug is used in the treatment of verapamil overdose?**

Calcium chloride.

O   **If a defibrillator is available, what is the immediate treatment of a patient with ventricular fibrillation?**

Unsynchronized countershock at 200J.

O   What is the differential diagnosis of pulseless electrical activity?

Tension pneumothorax, acidosis, MI, PE, OD, cardiac tamponade, hypoxia, hypovolemia, hyperkalemia, and hypothermia (TAMPOT plus 4H is the pnemonic).

O   What is the differential diagnosis of asystole?

Drug overdose, acidosis, hyperkalemia, hypothermia, hypokalemia, hypoxia.

O   A 28 year-old presents with hemodynamically stable paroxysmal supraventricular tachycardia (PSVT) at a rate of 170. What is the drug of choice?

Vagal maneuvers are tried first. If unsuccessful, adenosine is the drug of choice.

O   What is the treatment of choice for rapid atrial fibrillation in a patient with Wolff-Parkinson-White syndrome?

Cardioversion if the patient is unstable, otherwise procainamide (20 to 30 mg/min up to 17 mg/kg) is the treatment of choice. The infusion should be stopped if further widening of the QRS or hypotension occurs.

O   Permanent pacemakers have a coding system of 5 letters. The first letter refers to chamber paced, the second to chamber sensed. What does the third letter refer to?

Mode or Response. It comes in several flavors including I = Inhibited, T = Triggered, D = Double, R = Reverse and O = nOne.

O   What percentage of Americans experiencing cardiac arrest are resuscitated? What percentage of these suffer neurological damage?

Up to one-third are resuscitated and survive to discharge. Of this group, 20 to 40% develop permanent brain damage ranging from subtle to severe.

O   Tachycardia occurs after a cardiac arrest and is treated successfully with defibrillation and epinephrine. Would you treat this post-resuscitation rhythm?

If the patient has a pulse and is hemodynamically stable, no treatment may be necessary. If epinephrine is responsible for the tachycardia, it should resolve quickly. Sustained sinus tachycardia should not be allowed to persist, however, as it increases myocardial oxygen consumption.

O   T/F: An AICD (automated implantable cardioverter-defibrillator) is a contraindication to defibrillation.

False. If functioning, the AICD should assess, charge and shock within 30 seconds. If the patient is in ventricular fibrillation (VF) and a shock is not being delivered, proceed with external defibrillation.

O   Match the rhythm with the type of SVT.

1) Wolf-Parkinson-White syndrome
2) Multifocal atrial tachycardia
3) Atrial fibrillation
4) Atrial flutter
5) Accelerated junctional tachycardia
6) Unifocal atrial tachycardia
7) Intra-arterial reentrant tachycardia
8) Nodal tachycardia

a) AV reciprocating tachycardia
b) Automatic tachycardia
c) Reentrant atrial tachycardia
d) AV reentrant nodal tachycardia

Answers: (1) a, (2) b, (3) c, (4) c, (5) d, (6) b, (7) c, and (8) d.

O   What are the common causes of multifocal atrial tachycardia?

COPD, CHF, sepsis, and methylxanthine toxicity. Treat the arrhythmia with magnesium, verapamil, or beta-adrenergic agents.

O   What are some causes of SVT?

Digitalis toxicity, pericarditis, MI, COPD, pre-excitation syndromes, mitral valve prolapse, rheumatic heart disease, pneumonia, and ethanol.

O   What is the most common associated electrocardiographic abnormality found in patients with left anterior hemiblock on ECG?

LVH.

O   How does the P wave axis on the surface electrocardiogram help to differentiate between patients with chronic obstructive lung disease and restrictive lung disease?

A P wave axis of + 90 degrees is highly suggestive of chronic obstructive lung disease. Right axis deviation of the P wave is found in 80% of patients with chronic obstructive lung disease, but only in 7% of patients with restrictive lung disease. Conversely, 53% of patients with restrictive lung disease have a horizontal P wave axis, compared to only 8% of patients with chronic obstructive lung disease.

O   What is Ashman phenomenon and how does one detect it on ECG?

Ashman phenomenon is a form of aberrrant conduction and is a function of premature excitation due to altered duration of the refractory period. It usually exhibits RBBB morphology and may be associated with left anterior or, less commonly, left posterior fascicular block. It is suggested by the following: 1) a relatively long cycle immediately preceding the cycle terminated by the aberrant QRS complex, 2) RBBB aberrancy with normal orientation of the initial QRS vector, 3) irregular coupling of the aberrant QRS complex, and 4) lack of compensatory pause following the aberrant QRS complex.

O   What is acceleration-dependent aberrancy?

This form of aberrancy occurs at relatively slow rates, frequently below 75 beats/min. The aberrancy often depends on very small changes in cycle length and it persists at a longer cycle and normalization at a shorter cycle length that that which initiated the aberration.

O   How does acceleration-dependent aberrancy differ from the physiological aberrancy observed in a normal heart?

1.   Appearance of aberrancy at relatively slow heart rates.
2.   Predominance of LBBB morphology.
3.   Independence from the immediately preceding cycle length.
4.   Occasional appearance without or with only a slight change in cycle length.
5.   Association with heart disease.

O   What conditions, other than myocardial infarction, are Q waves seen?

The largest group of noninfarction Q waves is due to myocardial disease, including myocarditis, AIDS, cardiac amyloidosis, neuromuscular disorders such as progressive muscular dystrophy, scleroderma, postpartum myopathy, idiopathic cardiomyopathy, Friedreich's ataxia, myocardial replacement by tumor, anomalous coronary artery and coronary embolism. Noninfarction Q waves are common in hypertrophic cardiomyopathy, WPW, and LVH, and may also be seen in hypothermia, localized metabolic and electrolyte disturbances, COPD with or without cor pulmonle, pulmonary embolism and pneumothorax. Noninfarction Q waves may be transient or permanent and they occur as a result of a loss of electrophysiological function in the absence of irreversible cellular damage.

O   **What is the most common cause of a negative U wave on ECG?**

Hypertension. They may also be seen with aortic and mitral valve disease, RVH and myocardial ischemia.

O   **What is the most common reason for an abnormal electrocardiogram in an individual with no clinical heart disease?**

Limb lead reversal. It occurs commonly and may result in the erroneous diagnosis of arrhythmias, myocardial ischemia or infarction, ventricular hypertrophy or fascicular blocks. Lead reversal should be suspected when the limb leads exhibit significant changes while the precordial leads are normal and unchanged.

O   **How is lead reversal of the right and left arms manifested on the surface electrocardiogram?**

The so-called "mirror image" of lead I.

O   **How is lead reversal of the right leg and either arm lead manifested on the surface electrocardiogram?**

Lead II and III are isoelectric.

O   **What is the H-V interval and how does it relate to the P-R interval of the surface ECG?**

The H-V interval is the duration of electrical depolarization from the His bundle to the ventricular depolarization. A prolonged H-V interval, greater than 55 milliseconds, is associated with a greater likelihood of developing trifascicular block (rate of progression is slow-2 to 3 percent annually), having structural heart disease and higher mortality. Patients with a very long H-V interval (> 80-90 msec) are identified as having increased risk of developing high degree AV block.

O   **What is the sensitivity and specificity of an H-V interval for predicting the development of complete AV block?**

Specificity is 80%, but sensitivity is about 66%.

O   **What is the sinus node recovery time (SNRT) and what is its significance?**

The interval between the last paced high right atrial response and the first spontaneous (sinus) high right atrial response after termination of pacing is measured and is the sinus node recovery time (SNRT). Because spontaneous sinus rate influences the SNRT, the value is corrected by subtracting the spontaneous sinus node cycle length (prior to pacing) from the sinus recovery time. This is the corrected sinus node recovery time (CNSRT). Normal CSNRT values are generally less than 525 msec. Prolonged CSNRT has been found in patients suspected of having sinus node dysfunction. The range of normal for CSNRT less than 680 msec. The normal SNRT is less than 1600 msec.

O   **What is the sensitivity and specificity of the corrected sinus node recovery time for predicting sinus node dysfunction?**

The sensitivity is about 50-60 percent and the specificity is about 85-90 percent.

O   **How does the H-V interval differentiate SVT from VT?**

An SVT is recognized electrophysiologically by the presence of an H-V interval equaling or exceeding that recorded during normal sinus rhythm. In contrast, during ventricular tachycardia (VT), the H-V interval is shorter than normal, or more commonly, the His deflection cannot be recorded clearly.

❍   **What is the classification of heart rate and hemodynamic responses to head-up tilt table testing?**

Type I: Mixed
Heart rate rises initially and then falls, but the ventricular rate does not fall to less than 40 beats/min or falls to 40 beats/min for less than 10 seconds with or without asystole for less than 3 seconds.

Type IIA: Cardioinhibitory
Heart rate rises initially and then falls to a ventricular rate of less than 40 beats/min for greater than 10 seconds, or asystole occurs for greater than 3 seconds.

Blood pressure rises initially and then falls before heart rate falls.

Type IIB: Cardioinhibitory
Heart rate rises initially and then falls to a ventricular rate of less than 40 beats/min for greater than 10 seconds, or asystole occurs for greater than 3 seconds.

Blood pressure rises initially and only falls to hypotensive levels less than 80 mm Hg at or after the onset of rapid and severe heart rate fall.

Type III: Pure vasodepressor
Heart rate rises progressively and does not fall more than 10 per cent from peak at time of syncope.

Blood pressure falls to cause syncope.

VALVULAR HEART DISEASE

○ **What is the most frequent cause of mitral stenosis?**

Rheumatic fever. Far less common causes include congenital, malignant carcinoid, SLE, rheumatoid arthritis, infective endocarditis with a large vegetation, and the mucopolysaccharidoses of the Hunter-Hurley phenotype.

○ **What percentage of patients with rheumatic mitral stenosis are female?**

Two thirds.

○ **What percentage of patients with rheumatic heart disease have pure mitral stenosis?**

Twenty five percent. An additional 40% have combined MS and MR.

○ **What is the cross-sectional area of the mitral valve orifice in critical mitral stenosis?**

One cm^2 or less. The normal cross sectional area is between 4-6 cm^2. Mild mitral stenosis begins when the valve is reduced to approximately 2 cm^2.

○ **What are the principle symptoms in mitral stenosis?**

Dyspnea is most common. Patients with severe mitral stenosis can experience orthopnea, hemoptysis, chest pain, and frank pulmonary edema, often precipitated by exertion, fever, URI, sexual intercourse, pregnancy or the onset of rapid atrial fibrillation.

○ **What is Ortner's syndrome?**

Hoarseness caused by compression of the left recurrent laryngeal nerve by a greatly dilated left atrium, enlarged tracheobronchial lymph nodes, and dilated pulmonary arteries, occurring in severe, advanced mitral stenosis.

○ **What are the two most serious complications of mitral stenosis?**

Thromboembolism, most often occurring in the setting of atrial fibrillation, and pulmonary edema.

○ **What are the physical findings in patients with mitral stenosis?**

A low-pitched diastolic rumbling murmur, with or without a thrill, at the apex; a diminished S1 heart sound (may be virtually absent in severe MS); an opening snap following the second heart sound; a loud P2 heart sound in patients with pulmonary hypertension; fixed splitting of the second heart sound; a Graham Steell murmur of pulmonic regurgitation in patients with moderate to severe pulmonary hypertension; and a right parasternal S4 heart sound in patients with right heart failure.

○ **What maneuvers can one do to differentiate the opening snap of mitral stenosis from a split S2 sound?**

Sudden standing widens the A2-opening snap interval whereas a split S2 narrows on standing. Progressive narrowing of the A2-OS interval on serial examinations suggests an increase in the severity of mitral stenosis.

O   **What is the most accurate noninvasive technique for quantifying the severity of mitral stenosis?**

Doppler echocardiography.

O   **What is the medical management strategy of rheumatic mitral stenosis?**

Penicillin prophylaxis for beta-hemolytic streptococcal infections and prophylaxis for infective endocarditis, aggressive and prompt treatment of anemia and infections, avoidance of strenuous exertion, oral diuretics and sodium restriction in symptomatic patients, beta-blockers to reduce heart rate, cardioversion of atrial fibrillation if possible, aggressive slowing of refractory atrial fibrillation, and anticoagulant therapy in patients who have experienced one or more thromboembolic episodes or who have mechanical prosthetic valves.

O   **What is the asymptomatic period after an attack of rheumatic fever in patients with mitral stenosis?**

In temperate zones, such as the United States and Europe, about 15-20 years. In tropical and subtropical areas and in underdeveloped areas, about 6-12 years.

O   **What is the indication for mitral valve surgery or balloon valvuloplasty in patients with mitral stenosis?**

Moderate symptoms (Class II) or greater in a patient with moderate to severe mitral stenosis (mitral valve orifice size less than 1.0 cm^2 per square meter BSA-less than 1.5 to 1.7 cm^2 mitral valve area in normal-sized adults).

O   **A 28 year-old Hispanic female is referred to you for evaluation of dyspnea and palpitations. She has a diastolic murmur consistent with mitral stenosis. Echocardiography confirms severe, non-calcific mitral stenosis with trivial mitral regurgitation, with a mitral valve area of 0.8 cm^2. EKG reveals atrial fibrillation. She was recently married and would like to start a family. What is the most appropriate course of therapy for this patient?**

Open mitral valvotomy (commisurotomy) followed by cardioversion to normal sinus rhythm. This is palliative, obviates the need for anticoagulation for the immediate future, and results in at least 5-10 years of symptom free life for over half of patients.

O   **What is the complication and mortality rates for balloon mitral valvuloplasty?**

The reported mortality rate averages 0.5 %. Complications such as stroke and cardiac perforation occur in 1% of cases, atrial septal defect in 10%, and 2% develop severe mitral regurgitation requiring mitral valve replacement.

O   **What is the most common cause of mitral regurgitation?**

Rheumatic heart disease. It is more frequent in men than women. Other causes include infective endocarditis, mitral valve prolapse, ischemic heart disease, trauma, SLE, scleroderma, hypertrophic cardiomyopathy, dilated cardiomyopathy involving the left ventricle, and idiopathic degenerative calcification of the mitral annulus.

O   **What percentage of patients with coronary artery disease, considered for CABG, have mitral regurgitation?**

Thirty percent. It is secondary to ischemic papillary muscle dysfunction.

O   **What is the 5-year survival of medically treated patients with severe mitral regurgitation?**

Forty-five percent.

O   **What are the physical findings of patients with chronic mitral regurgitation?**

Harsh, pansystolic murmur heard best at the apex, radiating to the axilla or the base. The murmur is diminished by maneuvers that decrease preload or afterload, such as amyl nitrate inhalation, Valsalva or standing and increases with maneuvers that increase preload or afterload, such as squatting, handgrip or phenylephrine administration.

O   **What are the most common causes of acute mitral regurgitation?**

Acute myocardial infarction with papillary muscle dysfunction (15% of acute MI results in acute mitral regurgitation) or papillary muscle rupture (.3% of acute MI), infective endocarditis, chordae tendinae rupture secondary to chest trauma, rheumatic fever, mitral valve prolapse, and hypertrophic cardiomyopathy with rupture of chordae tendinae.

O   **What are the physical findings in patients with severe, chronic mitral regurgitation?**

Diminished S1 heart sound with wide splitting of S2, a loud P2 in patients with pulmonary hypertension, an S3 gallop at the apex, and a harsh pansystolic murmur at the apex with a thrill.

O   **Which is the best test to assess the detailed anatomy of rheumatic mitral valve disease and determine whether mitral valve replacement is necessary or whether reconstruction is feasible?**

Transesophageal echocardiography.

O   **What is the appropriate medical management of mitral regurgitation?**

Vasodilator therapy with ACE inhibitors is the hallmark of therapy, even in patients who are asymptomatic. Diuretics are used in patients with severe MR. Cardiac glycosides, such as digoxin, are indicated in patients with severe MR and clinical evidence of heart failure. Endocarditis prophylaxis is indicated in all patients with MR. Anticoagulation should be given to all patients in atrial fibrillation.

O   **A 33 year-old female comes to you for a physical and you notice a harsh systolic murmur at the apex that is also heard at the base. The murmur increases on standing and Valsalva and decreases with handgrip. What is the most likely finding on echocardiography?**

Mitral valve prolapse. The murmur of pure mitral regurgitation decreases with Valsalva and standing and increases with handgrip or squatting.

O   **A forty-six year-old male with a history of rheumatic fever at age 12 is admitted with an acute myocardial infarction. The patient's post-MI course is complicated by congestive heart failure. Echocardiogram reveals severe mitral regurgitation with rupture of one of the papillary muscles, prolapse of the posterior mitral valve leaflet without apparent calcification. Systolic function by echocardiogram is mildly reduced. What is the appropriate course of action in this patient?**

Mitral valve reconstruction and repair of the papillary muscle.

O   **What are the indications for operation in patients with severe, chronic mitral regurgitation?**

Patients with NYHA class II symptoms with end-systolic LV diameter of >45mm by echocardiography. Asymptomatic patients with severe MR under the age of 70 with ejection fractions less than 70% and end-systolic LV diameter >40mm by echocardiography who are likely to be candidates for mitral valve repair should also be strongly considered for surgery.

O   **What is the classic triad of symptoms of aortic stenosis?**

Syncope (often exertional), angina, and heart failure.

O   **What is the most common cause of aortic stenosis in patients under age 65?**

Calcification of congenitally bicuspid aortic valves (50%) followed by rheumatic heart disease (25%).

O   **What is the most common cause of aortic stenosis in patients over age 65?**

Calcific degeneration of the aortic leaflets.

O   **Once patients with aortic stenosis become symptomatic, what is their average survival without valve replacement?**

From the onset of syncope or angina, the mean survival is 2-3 years. From the onset of congestive heart failure, the mean survival is 1.5 years.

O   **A seventy-two year-old gentleman is referred to you by a general surgeon because of a systolic heart murmur. On examination, you hear a mid-systolic crescendo-decrescendo murmur at the right parasternal second ICS, radiating to the carotids. Carotid upstroke is delayed. The patient is asymptomatic without any history of angina or syncope. Echocardiography reveals an aortic valve area of 0.85 cm^2. He is not in need of elective surgery. What should you advise the patient to do?**

Surgery is not necessary at this point, but the patient should be told that he must report any symptoms of angina, dyspnea, or syncope. At that point, he should be promptly referred for left heart catheterization and coronary angiography in preparation for surgical replacement of the valve. In the meantime, repeat echocardiography should be carried out every 6-12 months.

O   **What is the operative risk for aortic valve replacement?**

In patients without frank CHF, the operative risk ranges from 2-8%. It is not appreciably higher in patients requiring concomitant myocardial revascularization.

O   **What is the strongest predictor of postoperative LV dysfunction following aortic valve replacement?**

Preoperative LV dysfunction

O   **How does a heart murmur reflect the severity of aortic stenosis?**

The longer the duration of the murmur and the greater the increase in intensity of the murmur, the more severe the aortic stenosis. The degree of "loudness" of the murmur is not as important in assessing severity.

O   **What is the best pharmacologic agent for patients with asymptomatic aortic stenosis?**

Without contraindications, beta-blockers are the best agents as they are the most useful in treating the left ventricular hypertrophy and its sequelae that develop as a result of aortic stenosis.

○   **A 68 year-old female with severe asymptomatic aortic stenosis suddenly complains of dyspnea and palpitations. On EKG, she is found to be in atrial fibrillation with a ventricular rate of 130 beats per minute. What is the most appropriate action to be taken?**

Immediate DC cardioversion followed by a search for previously unrecognized mitral valve disease. Once stabilized, the patient should be referred for cardiac catheterization and aortic valve replacement.

○   **What percentage of patients with mitral valve prolapse develop severe mitral regurgitation or infective endocarditis, requiring mitral valve surgery?**

About 5%, mostly men over the age of 50.

○   **What is the most common sustained tachyarrhythmia in patients with mitral valve prolapse?**

Paroxysmal supraventricular tachycardia.

○   **What do patients with mitral valve prolapse have in common with patients with recognized heritable disorders of connective tissue?**

Mitral valve prolapse may be inherited as an autosomal dominant phenotype and a large proportion of patients with mitral valve prolapse have systemic features such as anterior chest deformity, scoliosis, kyphosis, hypermobile joints and arm span greater than height. In addition, mitral valve prolapse is common in patients with Marfan's syndrome, the Ehlers-Danlos syndrome and adult polycystic kidney disease.

○   **What is mitral valve prolapse syndrome?**

A symptom complex consisting of palpitations, chest pain, easy fatigability, exercise intolerance, dyspnea, orthostatic phenomena, and syncope or pre-syncope in patients with mitral valve prolapse, predominantly related to autonomic dysfunction.

○   **What disorders are seen with increased frequency in patients with MVP syndrome?**

Graves' disease, asthma, migraine headaches, sleep disorders, fibromyositis, and functional gastrointestinal syndromes.

○   **What are the most beneficial therapies in patients with mitral valve prolapse?**

Daily exercise, beta-blockers, adequate intravascular volume and reassurance.

○   **What infrequent cause of mitral regurgitation is associated with an increased risk of stroke, independent of other factors?**

Mitral annular calcification.

○   **A 28 year-old black female comes to you with pain and stiffness in her shoulders, knees, elbows and wrists for three days. She is acutely febrile, but denies cough, shortness of breath, dysuria, diarrhea, abdominal pain. On auscultation, you notice a harsh pansystolic murmur at the apex radiating to the axilla. Prior to her symptoms, she felt well, but states that she has frequent episodes of joint pain which last a couple of days, then disappear. She denies any vaginal discharge and denies any sexual intercourse for the last 6 weeks. Her mother has rheumatoid arthritis. Her sedimentation rate is 50. What should you suspect and test for in this patient?**

The primary anti-phospholipid syndrome of SLE.

○   **What is the most common cause of isolated severe aortic regurgitation?**

Aortic root dilatation resulting from medial disease. Other common causes include congenital (bicuspid) aortic valve, previous infective endocarditis, and rheumatic heart disease.

O   **A 64 year-old gentleman who is three weeks post-cholecystectomy suffers from moderate malnutrition. He has been on TPN for 10 days and for the last four days, has spiked a fever of 102F. The patient is noticeably dyspneic with a respiratory rate of 26 and a HR of 110, in sinus rhythm by ECG. Blood cultures grow Candida albicans. CXR reveals moderate pulmonary congestion. An S3 gallop is heard at the apex and a low pitched decrescendo diastolic murmur is heard at the LSB. An echocardiogram reveals a 17 mm diameter vegetation on the non-coronary cusp of the aortic valve and Doppler echo reveals severe aortic regurgitation. What is the best course of action for this patient?**

IV Amphotericin, IV vasodilators such as Nitroprusside, and IV Dobutamine, followed by urgent AV replacement. Vegetations larger than 10 mm in diameter, particularly fungal, are rarely controlled with pharmacologic therapy alone, and surgery is almost always needed, even if the aortic regurgitation is mild or moderate.

O   **What are some of the physical findings in severe aortic regurgitation?**

Corrigan's pulse (abrupt distension of the peripheral pulse with quick collapse), Quincke's sign (capillary pulsations seen in the fingertips), de Musset's sign (headbobbing with each beat), bisferious pulse in the brachial or femoral pulse, Traube's sign ("pistol shot" systolic and diastolic sounds heard over the femoral artery, Muller's sign (systolic pulsations of the uvula, and Duroziez's sign (systolic murmur on proximal compression of the femoral artery and diastolic murmur on distal compression of the femoral artery. A wide pulse pressure is noted with persistence of Korotkoff sounds even to zero may be found. A hyperdynamic apical impulse with a decrescendo diastolic murmur at the LSB is noted.

O   **What murmur may be mistaken for mitral stenosis?**

The Austin-Flint murmur of severe aortic regurgitation which occurs from a powerful regurgitant jet from the aorta, imparted to the anterior leaflet of the mitral valve, limiting the opening of the anterior leaflet of the mitral valve.

O   **What is the survival of chronic aortic regurgitation after diagnosis?**

The five-year survival, after diagnosis, is 75%. The ten-year survival is 50%. Once symptoms begin, without surgical treatment, death occurs within 4 years after the development of angina, 2 years after the development of CHF.

O   **What percentage of patients with asymptomatic severe aortic regurgitation develop LV systolic dysfunction, sudden death or symptoms within 10 years?**

40%.

O   **What is the 5 and 10-year mortality of symptomatic severe aortic regurgitation without surgical valve replacement?**

25% and 50%, respectively.

O   **What are the indications for aortic valve replacement in patients with chronic aortic regurgitation?**

LV end-systolic dimension of >50mm, LVEF < 50%, and the onset of symptoms of angina or CHF.

O **What is the preferred pharmacologic agent in patients with asymptomatic chronic aortic regurgitation?**

Nifedipine, or ACE inhibitors. Both have shown major improvements in LVEF and major reduction in LV end-diastolic volume and mass with significantly lower incidence of the need for aortic valve replacement at 5 years.

O **What is the most common acquired abnormality that produces clinically significant tricuspid regurgitation?**

Dilatation of the tricuspid annulus related to right ventricular dilatation.

O **What is the most common congenital abnormality producing tricuspid regurgitation?**

Tricuspid valve prolapse. Less commonly is Ebstein's anomaly.

O **What is the most common cause of acute tricuspid regurgitation and what is the preferred management of this situation?**

Tricuspid valve endocarditis, often as a result of intravenous drug abuse. The preferred management is complete removal of the valve with immediate or eventual replacement of the valve. Antibiotic therapy usually is futile in preventing valve surgery.

O **A 38 year-old Hispanic female with known mitral valve prolapse is scheduled for dental cleaning. Her dentist calls you asking for recommendations for endocarditis prophylaxis. She is not allergic to penicillin. What are your recommendations?**

Amoxicillin 3.0 gms po one hour before the procedure followed by 1.5 gms po six hours after the initial dose.

O **What is the incidence of culture-negative endocarditis?**

About 5%.

O **How does the sensitivity of transthoracic echocardiography compare with transesophageal echocardiography in the diagnosis of infective endocarditis?**

Transthoracic echocardiography carries a diagnostic sensitivity of 30-40%, whereas transesophageal echocardiography carries a diagnostic sensitivity between 90-100%.

O **A 55 year-old gentleman who underwent a 4-vessel CABG three years ago and who has mild mitral and tricuspid regurgitation is scheduled for colonoscopy for rectal bleeding? What recommendations regarding endocarditis prophylaxis would you give the surgeon?**

No antibiotic prophylaxis is needed in this setting.

O **T/F: Osler's nodes are usually nodular and painful.**

True. In contrast, the macular Janeway lesions are painless.

O **What conditions, other than infective endocarditis, are associated with Osler's nodes?**

Nonbacterial thrombotic endocarditis, gonococcal infections and hemolytic anemia.

O **What organisms are most frequently implicated in endocarditis in intravenous drug abusers?**

Gram negative and fungal organisms.

O   **What is the most frequently reported bacterial isolate in patients with myocardial abscesses?**

Staphylococcus aureus.

O   **What is mural endocarditis?**

Inflammation and disruption of the nonvalvular endocardial surface of the cardiac chambers.

O   **What organisms are most frequently implicated in endocarditis in intravenous drug abusers?**

Gram negative and fungal organisms.

O   **What is the sensitivity of two-dimensional transesophageal echocardiograms for detecting vegetations?**

95%.

O   **Who is at high risk for developing endocarditis?**

People with prosthetic heart valves, previous incidents of endocarditis, complex congenital heart disease, intravenous drug use and surgically devised systemic pulmonary shunts.

O   **What patients have a moderate risk for developing endocarditis?**

Those with acquired valvular dysfunction, hypertrophic cardiomyopathy and uncorrected congenital heart defects.

O   **What is the most common organism associated with endocarditis?**

Streptococcus viridans.

O   **Fungi cause what percentage of prosthetic valve associated infective endocarditis?**

15%.

O   **History of contact with mammals and/or birds may suggest infection by what organisms?**

Coxiella burnetii (Q fever), *Brucella* species or *Chlamydia psittaci*.

O   **A nosocomial cluster of cases postoperatively may be caused by what organisms?**

Legionella or *Mycobacterium* species.

O   **What organism, once accounting for up to 25% of cases of endocarditis, is now only responsible for only 1 to 2% of cases?**

Neisseria gonorrhoeae.

O   **What is the appropriate treatment for patients with infective endocarditis?**

Intravenous antibiotics for 3 to 6 weeks and heparin/coumadin. Close follow-up is necessary and the patient should have a series of 2 separate negative blood cultures to demonstrate resolution of the condition.

○ **What is the etiology of idiopathic hypertrophic subaortic stenosis (IHSS)?**

A hypertrophic myopathy of the left ventricular outflow tract.

○ **What signs and symptoms are associated with myocardial abscesses?**

Low-grade fevers, chills, leukocytosis, conduction system abnormalities, nonspecific ECG changes and signs and symptoms of acute MI.

○ **What maneuvers will increase hypertrophic cardiomyopathy murmurs?**

Valsalva, standing, and amyl nitrate.

○ **What maneuvers will decrease hypertrophic cardiomyopathy murmurs?**

Handgrip, squatting, and leg elevation in the supine patient.

ATHEROSCLEROTIC VASCULAR DISEASE AND PERICARDIAL DISEASE

○ **Are aortic aneurysms more common in men or in women?**

Ten times more common in men. Other risk factors include hypertension, athersclerosis, diabetes, smoking, alcoholism, hyperlipidemia, syphillis, Marfan's disease, and Ehlers-Danlos disease.

○ **What is a true aortic aneurysm?**

True aneurysms involve a dilatation of all three layers of the aorta.

○ **Where are true aortic aneurysms most likely to occur, in the thoracic or abdominal aorta?**

Abdominal aorta, below the renal arteries, is most common. This is due to the decreasing diameter of the aorta, less elastin and more branches. Thus, greater turbulent flow with a higher systolic pressure exists in the abdominal aorta as compared with the thoracic aorta.

○ **A 68 year-old male with diabetes and a 60 pack-year history of smoking presents with sudden, severe substernal chest discomfort, radiating through to the interscapular area. BP is 150/80 mm Hg in the right arm and 135/65 mm Hg in the left arm. He complains of right arm numbness and weakness and you hear a II/IV diastolic murmur along the left sternal border. ECG reveals 1.5 mm ST elevation in the inferior leads. What is the diagnosis?**

Acute proximal thoracic aortic dissection, with involvement of the right coronary artery and brachiocephalic artery, as well as acute aortic regurgitation.

○ **In the patient described in the last question, what other life-threatening complication must one look for, both on auscultation and on CXR?**

Pericardial effusion with cardiac tamponade. Look for pericardial rub on auscultation and marked cardiomegaly on CXR. Pulsus paradoxus of >10 mm Hg is virtually diagnostic of cardiac tamponade in this setting.

○ **What CXR findings occur with a dissecting thoracic aortic aneurysm?**

Tortuosity of the proximal aorta with an enlarged aortic knob, mediastinal widening, pleural effusion (most common on the left), extension of the aortic shadow, displaced trachea to the right, cardiomegaly, and separation of the intimal calcification from the outer contour that is greater than 5 mm.

○ **What is the Stanford classification of aortic dissections defined and how are they treated?**

1) Type A: Involving the proximal thoracic aorta from root to the left subclavian artery (DeBakey I & II). This condition requires emergent surgery.
2) Type B: Involving the descending aorta, distal to the left subclavian artery (DeBakey III). Usually managed medically.

❍   **A 77 year-old male presents with acute onset of scrotal and testicular pain. You notice scrotal and groin ecchymosis. What is the diagnosis?**

A ruptured aortic or iliac artery aneurysm.

❍   **Where is an aortic dissection most likely to occur?**

Dissection involves intimal tears that are propagated by hematoma formation. Tears most commonly occur in the proximal ascending aorta (60%). 20% are found between the origin of the left subclavian and the ligamentum arteriosum in the descending aorta, 10% are found in the aortic arch, and 10% are found in the abdominal aorta distal to the renal arteries.

❍   **What is the definitive diagnostic procedure of choice for dissecting aortic aneurysms?**

Aortography.

❍   **When should surgery be advised for a non-dissecting thoracic aneurysm? For a non-dissecting abdominal aneurysm?**

A non-dissecting thoracic aneurysm should be resected if it is larger than 6 cm in diameter or has symptoms attributable to the aneurysm. Thoracic aneurysm enlarging under observation should also be resected. Non-dissecting abdominal aneurysms should be surgically resected if it is larger than 4 cm in diameter.

❍   **What is the prognosis for an untreated dissecting aortic aneurysm?**

Twenty five percent die within 24 hours, 50% die within one week, 75% percent die within one month and 90% die within 3 months. With surgical treatment, the 10 year survival is 50%; the five year survival is 75-80%. Redissection occurs in 25% within 10 years of the original dissection.

❍   **What is the most common complication of ascending thoracic aorta aneurysms?**

Aortic valve insufficiency.

❍   **Which age group is typically afflicted with Marfan's syndrome accompanied by aortic dissection?**

Individuals between 30-50. Aortic aneurysms, in general, occur most frequently in individuals between 60-80.

❍   **What are the typical features of Takayasu's arteritis?**

Early symptoms include fever, myalgias, arthralgias, weight loss and pain over inflamed vessels. Late symptoms are referable to occlusive changes and include transient ischemic attacks, strokes, arm fatigue, leg claudication and angina.

❍   **What are the laboratory markers for Takayasu's disease?**

An elevated erythrocyte sedimentation rate (ESR), leukocytosis and anemia of chronic disease.

❍   **What are the arteriographic findings of Takayasu's disease?**

Segmental dilatations, stenoses and occlusions.

○   **What is the treatment for patients with Takayasu's disease?**

Surgery is required for the treatment of aneurysmal and stenotic lesions with failure of medical management.

○   **What are the typical features of giant cell (temporal) arteritis?**

A flu-like prodrome with fever and malaise, weight loss, scalp tenderness, headache and myalgias. Pain over the temporal or occipital arteries, jaw claudication and eye symptoms follow.

○   **What are the most common causes of acute pericarditis?**

Idiopathic, infectious, neoplastic, radiation, uremia, myocardial infarction, autoimmune, rheumatologic, trauma, drugs and myxedema.

○   **What triad of findings confirms the diagnosis of pericarditis?**

Chest pain, pericardial friction rub and ECG abnormalities.

○   **What ECG changes are associated with pericarditis?**

ST elevation in at least 7 leads except V1 and aVR. PR segment depression may also be present.

○   **What is the treatment for acute pericarditis?**

Treatment of the underlying problem and non-steroidal anti-inflammatory agents. Steroids and narcotic analgesics may be required.

○   **What is the etiology of transient monocular blindness (amaurosis fugax) in patients with temporal arteritis?**

Occlusion of the terminal retinal arterioles from atherosclerotic emboli arising from the carotid bifurcation.

○   **What rheumatologic condition is frequently associated with temporal arteritis?**

Polymyalgia rheumatica.

○   **What is the appropriate management of Paget-Schroetter syndrome?**

Heparinization, direct infusion thrombolysis, thoracic outlet decompression and percutaneous angioplasty if residual venous stenosis exists. Venoplasty is occasionally required.

○   **What are the signs and symptoms of the subclavian steal syndrome?**

Dizziness, diplopia, ataxia, bilateral sensory or motor deficits or syncope when exercising the ipsilateral arm.

○   **What are the indications for patch closure of a carotid endarterectomy (CEA)?**

Patients with small arteries and re-do endarterectomies for recurrent stenosis.

○   **A 67 year-old male states that he had a 3-hour episode of left arm numbness and extreme weakness. The physical exam is significant for a right carotid bruit and a very subtle decrease in left**

grip strength. What is the appropriate management?

A head CT scan, without contrast, ECG, echocardiography and a carotid duplex study. Increasingly, experienced vascular surgeons proceed to endarterectomy without angiography in appropriate clinical situations.

○   **When should CEA be performed?**

Timing is determined by the size of the infarct, presence of hemorrhage and extent of neurologic deficit. Early anticoagulation is appropriate in patients with cardiac dysrhythmia or cerebral infarct without a hemorrhagic component.

○   **Which artery must frequently be divided to gain exposure to the hypoglossal nerve during CEA?**

The artery to the sternocleidomastoid muscle.

○   **What are the characteristics of fibromuscular dysplasia in the carotid artery?**

Alternating short intervals of dilatation and stenotic fibromuscular thickenings, turbulence with thromboembolic events, transient ischemic attacks, stroke and intracranial aneurysms.

○   **What are the clinical characteristics of chronic constrictive pericarditis?**

Progressive edema, ascites, hepatomegaly and exertional dyspnea.

○   **What is the treatment of choice for patients with constrictive pericarditis?**

Pericardiectomy.

○   **What are the risks and complications of pericardiocentesis?**

Cardiac tamponade, myocardial infarction, intra-abdominal injuries and pneumothorax.

○   **Following a high-speed motor vehicle accident (MVA), evaluation reveals a widened mediastinum. What is the pathophysiology of the probable injury?**

The ligamentum arteriosum tethers the under surface of the aortic arch to the proximal left main pulmonary artery, at a point just distal to the left subclavian artery. Sudden deceleration causes shearing between the mobile aortic arch and the immobile descending aorta, resulting in aortic disruption.

○   **What are the typical symptoms of anterior circulation cerebrovascular ischemia?**

Aphasia, contralateral weakness or sensory change in the upper or lower extremities and contralateral facial droop.

○   **What clinical symptoms are most typical of vertebrobasilar ischemia?**

Diplopia, dizziness, syncope, dysarthria, ataxia and bilateral extremity sensory change or weakness.

○   **What is the mortality rate for patients requiring permanent anticoagulation therapy?**

1 to 2% per year.

○   **Following an MVA where the patient was wearing a shoulder strap, the only notable physical findings are left neck tenderness with mild ecchymosis and a brief episode of aphasia reported by**

rescue workers at the scene. A duplex carotid Doppler study reveals a small intimal flap in the distal common carotid artery. What is the most appropriate management of this patient?

Surgical repair.

○   **What is the initial mainstay of medical therapy in all types of acute aortic dissection?**

Intensive continuous monitoring. Cardiac output and blood pressure must be promptly reduced to as low a level as possible while still maintaining end organ perfusion. Sodium nitroprusside is the first line antihypertensive agent (infused at 1 to 2 mcg/kg/min to maintain systolic blood pressure at 90 to 100 mm Hg or lower, if needed for pain control). Simultaneous intravenous beta blockade with esmolol is administered to prevent tachycardia and maintain a heart rate less than 70.

○   **During CEA, what hemodynamic changes may occur with manipulation of the carotid bulb?**

Bradycardia and hypotension.

○   **What is the treatment for these hemodynamic changes?**

Injection of 1 or 2 cc of 1% plain lidocaine into the carotid bulb periadventitial tissue. Systemic atropine may be considered for persistent intraoperative bradycardia. Postoperative bradycardia may be treated with judicious administration of atropine in the symptomatic patient. Occasionally, low dose infusion of Neo-Synephrine is needed to maintain an appropriate mean arterial pressure.

○   **With respect to CEA, what intraoperative measures minimize the risk of perioperative stroke?**

Smooth induction of anesthesia, avoidance of hemodynamic instability and resultant low cerebral blood flow, meticulous dissection of the carotid artery with minimal manipulation, selective shunting, appropriate flushing and back-bleeding of the arteries, anticoagulation and meticulous closure.

○   **What are the 3 types of recurrent carotid stenosis?**

Myointimal hyperplasia, recurrent atherosclerotic lesions and residual plaque left from the primary operation.

○   **Other than arch aortography, what diagnostic tests may be helpful in ruling out traumatic aortic disruption?**

Transesophageal echocardiography and spiral CT scan of the chest.

○   **What are the risks of pericardiocentesis?**

Hemothorax, pneumothorax, hemorrhage from myocardial or coronary artery laceration and tamponade from this hemorrhage.

○   **What is the most common location of a recurrent carotid stenosis?**

At the previous endarterectomy site.

○   **What are the cardiovascular variables associated with aortic cross clamping at the infrarenal level?**

Minimal changes. There is a 2% increase in mean arterial pressure (MAP), no change in the left ventricular end-diastolic pressure (LVEDP) and a reduction in the ejection fraction (EF) of 3%.

○   **What are the determinants of cerebral blood flow during carotid endarterectomy (CEA)?**

Partial pressure of arterial CO2 and O2 (PaCO2 and PaO2), arterial blood pressure, autoregulation, venous blood pressure, anesthetic drugs, metabolic factors (seizures, shivering) and pain.

○   **How is the stump pressure used in CEA?**

It is dependent upon extracranial collateral flow, systemic pressure and cerebrovascular resistance. Pressures of 50 to 60 mm Hg are thought to indicate adequate flow. However, the correlation between EEGs and stump pressure is less than good, since flow does not necessarily indicate adequate perfusion.

○   **What is the most common cause of late failure of reversed saphenous vein grafts?**

Atherosclerosis.

○   **What is the most common site for atherosclerotic occlusion in the lower extremities?**

The distal superficial femoral artery.

○   **What is the most common etiologic factor involved in ascending aortic aneurysms?**

Cystic medial necrosis.

○   **What is the expected ankle-brachial index (ABI) in patients with intermittent claudication?**

Between 0.5 and 0.8.

○   **What are the Doppler signs of acute DVT?**

Absence of flow in a vein segment, continuous (non phasic) flow distal to an obstruction, lack of augmentation proximal to an obstruction and increased flow in the superficial veins.

○   **Repair of which type of aneurysm is associated with the highest operative mortality rate?**

Transverse aortic arch aneurysms.

○   **How accurate is a ventilation/perfusion (V/Q) scan in diagnosis of an acute pulmonary embolus (PE)?**

Pulmonary angiography has shown that in a patient with a high probability V/Q scan, the incidence of PE is 87%. With an intermediate probability reading, the incidence is 30% and with a low probability reading, the incidence is 14%.

○   **What are the indications for an emergency pulmonary embolectomy?**

Persistent refractory hypotension despite maximal resuscitation in a patient with a documented acute massive PE.

○   **What is the natural history of valvular reflux after an acute DVT?**

Valvular reflux develops progressively from the time of acute DVT.

○   **What is the appropriate treatment for a 30 year-old male with an asymptomatic 3 cm splenic artery aneurysm?**

Surgical repair of the aneurysm.

○   **What is the treatment of choice for acute arterial embolus to the lower extremity?**

Intravenous heparin (a 5,000 or 10,000 unit bolus) followed by continuos intravenous administration.

○   **What is the diagnostic test of choice for venous or arterial disease?**

Doppler ultrasonography with B-mode ultrasonography.

○   **What is the contraindication to thromboendarterectomy?**

Concomitant aneurysmal disease.

○   **What is the initial pathophysiologic event in the development of atherosclerosis?**

Platelet adherence.

○   **What is the appropriate treatment for "subclavian steal" syndrome?**

Carotid-subclavian bypass or axillo-axillary bypass.

○   **What is the treatment of choice for patients with Leriche syndrome?**

Aortoiliac-bifemoral bypass.

○   **What are the prerequisites for success of a cross-femoral venous bypass for relief of symptoms due to a chronically occluded iliac vein?**

Patency of the contralateral iliofemoral and caval runoff, presence of a supine resting pressure gradient in excess of 4 to 5 mm Hg between the femoral veins in the involved and contralateral limbs and a good quality contralateral saphenous vein.

○   **What is the appropriate management of reperfusion injury following vascular repair?**

Serum electrolyte evaluation and intravenous administration of sodium bicarbonate and mannitol.

○   **T/F: Patients with a carotid bruit are at increased risk of stroke during abdominal surgery.**

False.

○   **What is the appropriate management of a 47 year-old woman with chronic lymphedema?**

Elevation of the legs, compression stockings when ambulating, periodic compression pumps for severe cases and manual lymph drainage.

○   **What is the treatment of choice for a patient with unilateral aortoiliac occlusion and an intra-abdominal infection?**

Femoral-femoral crossover graft.

○   **T/F: Impedance plethysmography (IPG) is less accurate than duplex scanning for detection of chronic DVT.**

True.

○   **What is the most common cause of arterial mycotic aneurysms?**

Use of prosthetic graft material.

❍   **What is the appropriate treatment of a patient with symptomatic carotid stenosis on the right and asymptomatic 50% stenosis on the left?**

CEA on the symptomatic side only.

❍   **What are the characteristic symptoms of vertebral basilar ischemia?**

Diplopia, dysarthria, vertigo and tinnitus.

❍   **What are the indications for tibioperoneal bypass grafts?**

Gangrene of the forefoot, rest pain, necrotizing infection or a nonhealing wound.

❍   **What is the most common operative approach to AAA repair?**

Endoaneurysmal.

❍   **What are the alternatives to intra-arterial contrast angiography?**

Duplex examination, intraarterial ultrasound, CT angiography, MRA and angioscopy.

❍   **How is carotid arterial stenosis measured from an arteriogram?**

By comparing the diameter of the stenotic area with the diameter of the nondiseased distal internal carotid artery. This ratio is subtracted from one and expresses the percentage of diameter reduction.

❍   **What is the success rate of angioplasty for the following anatomic sites: iliac, femoral, popliteal and tibial?**

At 5 years, iliac angioplasty with stenting has a 90% success rate, 60% without a stint. Femoral-popliteal success rates approximate 30% at 5 years and tibial lesions are considerably lower.

❍   **What are the characteristics of fibromuscular dysplasia (FMD)?**

Eccentric stenoses with intervening areas of dilatation.

❍   **What is the major concern in a patient who develops bloody diarrhea following AAA repair?**

Ischemic colitis.

❍   **What is the leading cause of late death after aortic reconstruction?**

CAD.

❍   **What is the treatment of choice for patients with FMD?**

Percutaneous transluminal angioplasty (PTA).

❍   **What type of aortic aneurysm is associated with Marfan's syndrome?**

Type A.

○ **What causes the blood pressure fluctuation commonly seen after carotid surgery.**

Manipulation of the carotid body.

○ **What is the appropriate management for a 23 year-old male smoker who presents with symptoms of upper extremity ischemia?**

Patients with Buerger's disease are encouraged to quit smoking and are managed with analgesics.

○ **What is the treatment of choice for patients with superior vena cava (SVC) syndrome caused by malignancy?**

Radiation therapy.

○ **What are the causes of reduced urine output after aortic reconstructive procedures?**

Inadequate circulating blood volume, low cardiac output (CO), renal ischemia, acute tubular necrosis (ATN) and a kinked or clogged Foley catheter.

○ **What are the benefits of CEA versus antiplatelet agents in symptomatic carotid disease?**

CEA produces a 7-fold reduction in the long-term risk of stroke.

○ **What is the recurrence rate of ipsilateral internal carotid stenosis following CEA?**

10 to 15%.

○ **What is the treatment of choice for symptomatic thoraco-abdominal aneurysms?**

Intraluminal graft placement.

○ **What is the characteristic gross appearance of an inflammatory AAA?**

An intense, thick, white fibroplastic reaction with adherence to the third and fourth portions of the duodenum and the inferior vena cava (IVC).

○ **What is the most common cause of cerebral ischemia?**

Arterial emboli, most commonly from the aorta.

○ **What is the appropriate treatment for infected prosthetic grafts?**

Antibiotics, removal of the prosthesis and re-establishment of vascular continuity.

○ **What percentage of patients with traumatic thoracic aortic aneurysms survive long enough for a false aneurysm to develop?**

2%.

○ **What should be done for a patient who awakens with a new ipsilateral neurologic deficit following CEA?**

Bedside duplex, angiogram and/or re-exploration.

○ **What noninvasive tests are used to assess the severity of claudication?**

Resting segmental pressures and pulse-volume recordings may demonstrate occlusive disease. A graded-treadmill protocol will quantify the distance the patient can walk and demonstrate the typical pressure drop at the ankle following exercise.

○   **What is the contraindication to PTA?**

Intimal dissection (with occlusion, rupture or distal embolization).

○   **What factors result in an intraoperative increase in central venous pressure (CVP)?**

Hypervolemia, positive pressure ventilation, Trendelenberg positioning, right ventricular failure, biventricular failure, tricuspid valvular disease, pulmonary hypertension and emboli.

○   **What are the immediate postoperative concerns following CEA?**

CVA, intracerebral hemorrhage, hypertension, hypotension, hematoma, airway obstruction, injury to the recurrent laryngeal, superior laryngeal, hypoglossal or submandibular nerve and vascular headaches.

○   **What is the success rate for percutaneous transluminal angioplasty (PTA) of the iliac arteries?**

95%.

○   **What is the most common complication following AAA repair in a 60 year-old male?**

Impotence.

○   **What is the screening test of choice for carotid stenosis?**

Duplex scanning.

○   **What is the most common etiology of advanced venous insufficiency?**

Venous valvular incompetence.

○   **What is the most common symptom of acute pericarditis?**

Sharp or stabbing retrosternal or precordial chest pain. Pain increases when supine and decreases when sitting-up and leaning forward. Pain may be increased with movement and deep breaths. Other symptoms include fever, dyspnea described as pain with inspiration, and dysphagia.

○   **What physical findings are associated with acute pericarditis?**

Pericardial friction rub is the most common. Rub is best heard at the left sternal border or apex in a sitting leaning forward position. Other findings include fever and tachycardia.

○   **What ECG changes are seen in acute pericarditis?**

ST segment elevation in the precordial leads, especially V5 and V6 and in lead I. PR depression is seen in leads II, aVF, V4-V6.

○   **What percentage patients with angiogram proven pulmonary embolism have an initial ventilation-perfusion scan reported as low probability.**

12%!

O   **What are the most common symptoms and signs of PE?**

CP (88%).
Tachypnea (92%).
Dyspnea (84%).
Anxiety (59%).
Fever (43%).
Tachycardia (44%).
DVT (32%).
Hypotension (25%).
Syncope (13%).

O   **Can a patient with a PE have a PaO_2 greater than 90 mmHg?**

About 5% have a $PaO_2 > 90$ mmHg.

O   **What is the most common CXR finding in PE?**

Elevated dome of one hemidiaphragm as a result of decreased lung volume observed in 50% of all cases of pulmonary embolism. Other common findings include pleural effusions, atelectasis, and pulmonary infiltrates.

O   **What are two relatively specific findings in PE on CXR?**

Hampton's Hump - Area of lung consolidation with a rounded border facing the hilum.
Westermark's sign - Dilated pulmonary outflow tract ipsilateral to the emboli with decreased perfusion distal to the lesion.

O   **What does a normal perfusion scan rule out?**

Rules out a PE. An abnormal scan can be caused by PE, asthma, emphysema, bronchitis, pneumonia, pleural effusion, carcinoma, CHF, and atelectasis.

O   **What does normal ventilation with decreased perfusion suggest?**

PE.

O   **What are some of the indications for pulmonary angiography in a patient thought to have a PE?**

1. Patients at high risk for bleeding complications with anticoagulation.
2. Negative test for DVT and low or medium probability lung scans.
3. Unstable patients for whom fibrinolytic therapy is being considered.

O   **What are the typical arterial blood gas (ABG) changes associated with an acute PE?**

Hypoxemia and hypocarbia.

O   **What are the characteristic symptoms of Leriche syndrome?**

Bilateral lower extremity weakness, symmetrical atrophy, pallor of the legs and feet and inability to maintain an erection.

O   **What complications are associated with heparin administration?**

Bleeding, heparin induced thrombocytopenia and hypersensitivity reactions. Chronic heparin use is associated with osteoporosis, alopecia and hypoadrenalism.

O   **What are the indications for axillofemoral bypass?**

Infected aortic aneurysm, infected aortic prosthetic graft and patients who are at excessive risk for abdominal procedures.

O   **What is the most common origin of dissecting aneurysms?**

The ascending aorta.

O   **What is the mechanism of action of Coumadin?**

It inhibits the vitamin K-dependent coagulation factors (II, VII, IX and X).

O   **What are the major side effects of Coumadin?**

Bleeding, skin necrosis and neural tube birth defects.

O   **What are the complications of iliofemoral venous thrombectomy?**

PE, early re-thrombosis and wound complications.

O   **What is a papaverine test?**

When injected directly into a peripheral artery, papaverine causes a temporary increase in flow to the limb. The presence of significant stenosis proximal to the injection point will cause a sudden, temporary decrease in the intraarterial pressure measured below that point.

O   **What are the major indications for infrarenal vena cava filter placement?**

Documented lower extremity deep vein thrombosis (DVT) or PE with a recognized contraindication to anticoagulation, PE despite adequate anticoagulation, bleeding complications of anticoagulation and after pulmonary embolectomy.

O   **What are the most common complications of prosthetic arterial grafts?**

Fibrous hyperplasia, infection, graft failure and formation of false aneurysms.

O   **What is the most important factor contributing to flow through a stenotic artery?**

Diameter of the stenosis.

O   **What complications are associated with use of a Greenfield filter?**

Failure of insertion, incomplete opening, leg asymmetry, perforation of the inferior vena cava (IVC), hematoma at the insertion site, filter movement, recurrent PE and caval thrombosis.

O   **What is the most common site of occlusion from cardioarterial emboli?**

The common femoral artery.

O   **What factors contribute to the development of primary varicose veins?**

Valvular incompetence, weakness of the vein wall and presence of multiple arteriovenous fistulae.

○   **What is the most common site of origin of traumatic thoracic aorta aneurysms?**

Just distal to the origin of the left subclavian vein.

○   **What are the indications for surgical treatment of varicose veins?**

Leg pain, edema, episodes of recurrent thrombophlebitis and cosmesis.

○   **What are the criteria for diagnosis of lower extremity claudication?**

Leg pain with exertion, relieved by rest and elevation, ipsilateral iliac vein obstruction, venous hypertension at rest and elevation of venous pressure with exercise.

○   **What is the most common vasospastic disorder affecting women less than 40 years of age?**

Raynaud's disease/phenomenon.

○   **What is the relationship between the finding of a carotid bruit on physical examination and the degree of carotid stenosis?**

Almost none.

○   **What is the typical early presentation of a patient with acute mesenteric ischemia?**

Severe, generalized abdominal pain with a remarkably benign abdominal exam. There may also be nausea, vomiting or diarrhea.

○   **What is the typical presentation of a patient with chronic mesenteric ischemia?.**

Intermittent post-prandial epigastric pain that begins 30 to 60 minutes after eating and may persist for a few hours.

○   **T/F: The absence of a Doppler signal indicates the absence of flow?**

False.

○   **What diseases are associated with occlusive tibioperoneal atherosclerosis?**

Diabetes mellitus and Buerger's disease.

○   **What are the most common complications of arteriography?**

Renal failure, allergic reaction to contrast media, hematoma, pseudoaneurysm and arteriovenous fistulae.

○   **What is the natural history of claudication?**

Fewer than 10% of patients with claudication will progress to critical ischemia or amputation. Most of those who do progress have uncontrolled risk factors, diabetes mellitus and those who continue to smoke.

○   **What are the characteristic radiologic signs of aortic injury?**

Widening of the mediastinum, blunting of the aortic knob, left apical capping, deviation of the trachea to the right and depression of the left main bronchus.

❍   **What are the medical and behavioral treatments for claudication?**

Management of risk factors is essential (i.e., cessation of smoking and control of diabetes, hyperlipidemia and blood pressure are the initial maneuvers). A supervised time-based walking exercise program, especially in the absence of smoking, will build collaterals, lessen symptoms and increase walking tolerance. Trental may increase walking distance in some individuals with claudication.

❍   **What are the requirements for successful arterial reconstruction?**

Adequate inflow, adequate outflow and an adequate conduit.

❍   **What is the tri-modal distribution of graft failure?**

Technical error, intimal hyperplasia and progression of atherosclerotic disease.

❍   **How does the location of the distal anastomosis relate to graft patency?**

In general, the more distal the anastomosis, the lower the graft patency.

❍   **What is a pseudoaneurysm?**

An enlargement of a vascular circuit lacking the full layers of the vessel wall.

❍   **What is the difference between saccular and fusiform aneurysms?**

The usual aortic aneurysm is fusiform, where the dilation involves the entire circumference of the vessel. Many visceral and cerebral aneurysms are saccular, where the majority of the vessel circumference may be normal in caliber with only a portion of the circumference weakening and dilating.

❍   **What is the natural history of popliteal artery aneurysms?**

It tends to thrombose acutely and cause limb-threatening ischemia.

❍   **What is the relationship of a popliteal aneurysm to an AAA?**

Approximately 20% of patients with an AAA may have a popliteal aneurysm. 40 to 60% of patients with a unilateral popliteal aneurysm may have an AAA.

❍   **What is the thoracic outlet?**

The thoracic outlet is an anatomic structure formed by the first rib, clavicle and scalene muscles through which pass the brachial plexus, subclavian artery and subclavian vein. The nerves and artery are posterior to the vein and separated by the anterior scalene muscle.

❍   **What is thoracic outlet syndrome?**

Anything that narrows the outlet, such as muscular hypertrophy, fibrous tissue, scar tissue or fracture callus, can impinge on one or more of the structures within the thoracic outlet and cause symptoms.

❍   **What patients are at increased risk for DVT?**

Those with hypercoagulable body chemistries, previous DVT, lower-extremity trauma, orthopedic surgery, major pelvic operations, immobility, acute MI, CHF, malignancies and those taking oral contraceptives, especially if they smoke.

○ **What are the effective prophylactic measures for DVT?**

Coumadin, unfractionated heparin, low-molecular weight heparins, dextran, antiplatelet drugs such as aspirin or ticlid and sequential venous compression stockings (SCD's).

○ **Where is the most common site of peripheral aneurysms that develop from arteriosclerosis?**

The popliteal artery. Other sites include the femoral, carotid, and subclavian arteries.

○ **How long can ST and T changes persist after an episode of pain in unstable angina?**

Several hours.

○ **What is the most common symptom of aortic dissection?**

Interscapular back pain.

○ **Where do aortic dissections most often occur?**

Proximal ascending aorta (60%). Twenty percent of aortic dissections are found between the origin of the left subclavian and the ligamentum arteriosum in the descending aorta, and 10% are found in the aortic arch or the abdominal aorta. Dissection involves intimal tears propagated by hematoma formation.

○ **What aortic aneurysm diameter is generally considered to be an indication for surgery: a) in the thorax and b) in the abdomen?**

Those with non-dissecting thoracic aneurysm larger than 7 cm in diameter are candidates for surgery. However, surgery should be considered with smaller aneurysms for those with Marfan's syndrome, because of a higher incidence of rupture. Non-dissecting abdominal aortic aneurysms larger than 4 cm in diameter should be considered for surgical repair.

○ **A patient is brought in to the emergency room and is extremely lethargic. History obtained from a family member reveals that just prior to the patients change in mental status he complained of sharp and tearing chest pain beginning retrosternally and going to the back. The patient then lost consciousness. On physical exam the pulse is 110, the hear sounds are distant and the patient is extremely lethargic. All pulses are palpable and no murmurs appreciated. Neurological exam reveals no focal deficits. What is most likely cause of the patient's syncope?**

The patient's history and presentation is strongly suggestive of aortic dissection. Syncope without focal neurological findings in this patient is strongly suggestive of aortic dissection resulting in cardiac tamponade. In one recorded series of patients, syncope without neurological findings occurred in 6 of 124 patients. In each case there was evidence of rupture of the dissection into the pericardial cavity.

○ **A 68 year-old man with a history of hypertension and coronary artery disease presents to the emergency room with complaints of sudden onset of severe pain beginning in the mid scapular region. The pain was very intense at onset and has not changed. Physical exam revealed a blood pressure of 180/180, pulses are equal throughout and the patient is in moderate distress. Chest x-ray reveals mildly increased mediastinum. Electrocardiogram shows left ventricular hypertrophy but is otherwise unremarkable. You suspect aortic dissection, what is the most likely point of origin for the dissection?**

The site of origin for this dissection is most likely distal. Although pain may be felt simultaneously in the anterior and posterior chest with both proximal and distal dissections the lack of anterior pain in this patient suggests a distal site of origin. Conversely, the absence of inter-scapular pain generally implies a non-distal dissection, since 90% of patients with distal dissection do report back pain.

The presentation of this patient is also significant in that the patient had severe chest pain without ECG changes. This is very helpful in differentiating acute MI from aortic dissection.

O   **A 65 year-old woman with a history of hypertension presents to the emergency department complaining of severe onset of retrosternal chest pain radiating to the back and then down towards the abdomen. Physical exam reveals a blood pressure of 190/105, pulse 88 and regular, and the patient is in moderate distress. Physical exam is remarkable for the absence of a murmur and palpable pulses that are equal throughout. Electrocardiographic findings are remarkable and chest x-ray reveals a wide mediastinum. You diagnose aortic dissection and place the patient on nitroprusside. The patient's blood pressure decreases to 170/100 and she still complaints of some pain. You add labetalol to the regimen and the blood pressure further decreases to 160/100 with a decrease in pulse from 88 to 75bpm. Despite increasing doses of labetalol you are unable to get control of the pressure. What is the most likely explanation for this?**

Refractory hypertension can follow occlusion of one of both of the renal arteries. This results in the release of large amounts of renin. In this circumstance, intravenous use of ace inhibitors may be very effective in reducing the blood pressure. It should also be noted that the use of calcium channel blockers, in particular, Nifedipine, has also been used effectively in refractory hypertension associated with aortic dissection.

O   **What is the most common caused of occlusive peripheral vascular disease (PVD)?**

Atherosclerosis. The lower extremities are most frequently involved, but disease of the origin of the left subclavian artery is not uncommon.

O   **What is the most common symptom of occlusive PDV?**

Claudication. This is pain in the extremities with walking, and is relieved by rest. This must be distinguished from "Pseudoclaudication", which causes lower extremity pain with erect posture (Standing and walking). The latter is most often caused by lumbar spinal stenosis.

O   **What is "rest pain"?**

This is a severe pain resulting from progressive occlusive arterial disease. The pain is usually worse at night and the patient may hang the ischemic limb over the bed to get relief.

O   **Does the degree of intensity of a bruit heard on physical exam correlate with the degree of obstruction in occlusive vascular disease?**

No, there is no good correlation between intensity of the bruits and degree of obstruction. However, most bruits of occlusive arterial disease are systolic. If the bruits extend into diastole, then frequently the stenosis is greater than 80%.

O   **Does the absence of the dorsalis pedis pulse diagnose PVD?**

No. Absence of one or both dorsalis pedis pulse occurs in approximately 12% of normal patients. Of note, the posterior tibial artery is virtually always present in healthy people, and the absence of this pulse is an excellent indicator of occlusive peripheral arterial disease.

O   **A 68 year-old woman with obesity and hypertension consults you for an ulcer of the leg. She denies trauma, and states that it is not painful, but it will not heal. Physical exam reveals decreased distal pulses, and a shaggy lesion on the medial aspect of her right leg distally. The skin around it is pigmented and it is non tender. What is the most likely diagnosis?**

Venous stasis ulcer. The description is classic for Venous ulceration. Pain in the ulcer may occur, but when only superinfection is present.

○   **A 75 year-old with a history of hypertension, smoking, and coronary artery disease complains of a painful ulcer in his heal. It has been there for several months, and it will not heal. He states that he noticed it after slipping on a stair and striking his heal strongly on the step below. Physical examination reveals markedly reduced pulses with a discrete ulcer. What is the diagnosis?**

The patient's history and physical findings suggest occlusive peripheral vascular disease and the lesion is very characteristic of an ischemic ulcer. Other characteristics of these lesions include: a discrete ulcer edge, a pale ulcer base with or without eschar, and atrophic or inflamed surrounding skin. This lesion can be distinguished from a neurotrophic ulcer, which is painless, occurs in a similar distribution, but frequently is spontaneous at onset, rather than associated with trauma.

○   **What is the best method of evaluating PVD?**

Arteriography. This modality provides the most information on location and degree of occlusion, and the condition of the proximal and distal circulation. However, it is not generally necessary for diagnosis, which can frequently be made by history, physical exam and non-invasive studies. MR angiography is also an excellent modality for diagnosing and defining the extent of PVD.

○   **What is the most common cause death in patients with PVD?**

Coronary and cerebral arterial disease. Most patients with PVD will not die of their disease, and therapy directed specifically at their PVD will not improve life expectancy.

○   **What is the best predictor of limb survival in patients with occlusive PVD?**

In non-diabetic patients, symptoms are probably most reliable. Asymptomatic patients or those with only intermittent claudication have a rate of about 54% limb loss at 5 years. When most severe symptoms, rest pain, or ischemic ulceration is present, limb loss is significantly higher. Prognosis for both survival and limb loss is worse in diabetic patients.

○   **What are the main management options for intermittent claudication?**

Walking programs, Pharmacological therapy, and/or restoration of pulsatile blood flow. It should be noted that medical therapy generally implies cessation of smoking and avoidance of limb trauma as well as the use of pentoxifylline (Trental), which may improve walking distance in some patients. Unfortunately, presently available vasodilators have not been proven effective.

○   **What are the main forms of therapy employed to restore pulsatile flow?**

Arterial bypass surgery and percutaneous transluminal angioplasty. In general, the latter gives comparable long and short term results to surgery when "ideal" lesions are present. Arterial surgery is more often applied when disease is present in multiple locations.

○   **List 3 types of PVD not confined to the lower extremities.**

1. Thromboangiitis obliterans (Buerger's disease); 2. Connective tissue disease-related arteritis; 3. Giant cell arteritis.

○   **Buerger's disease affects which limbs most commonly?**

The lower extremities. Patients are typically male, less than 30 years of age at symptom onset and heavy smokers. The disease affects small and medium arteries and veins of both the upper and lower extremities. Treatment is non-invasive and disease activity will stop with cessation of tobacco use.

○   **What are the classic signs and symptoms of acute peripheral arterial occlusion?**

Pain, pallor, paraesthesia, pulselessness, and paralyses. Frequently, the presentation is more subtle, with complaints limited to coldness or paraesthesia of the affected extremity.

O   **What are the mechanisms of acute peripheral arterial occlusion?**

Embolization and thrombosis. Definitive therapy depends upon the nature of the acute occlusion, but in general heparin therapy should be initiated to protect collateral circulation. Conditions suggesting embolic mechanisms include congestive heart failure, atrial fibrillation, recent myocardial infarction, proximal atheromatous disease of arterial aneurysm.

Conditions suggesting thrombotic mechanisms include prior symptomatic PVD, active arteritis, acute aortic dissection and myeloproliferative disease.

O   **72 year-old man with a history of exertional chest pain complains of pain in both feet for 3 days. He says the pain is quite severe and noticed that one of this toes has turned blue. He also has noticed generalized bluish mottling of his lower extremities in a reticular pattern A cardiac catheterization performed one week ago revealed 2-vessel coronary artery disease. What is the patient's diagnosis?**

Atheroembolic disease (perhaps "cholesterol emboli syndrome"). The skin changes described are consistent with Livedo Reticularis and support diagnosis, as do the pain and blue toe. The recent cardiac catheterization is also strongly suggestive of this entity. Treatment includes aspirin or persantine, not heparin or coumadin.

O   **How does one distinguish primary from secondary Raynaud's phenomenon?**

Age at onset is approximately 40 for both, but primary usually affects females, is bilateral, symmetrical, and it involves the toes. Secondary usually effects males, may be bilateral but is not symmetrical and it does not involve the toes. The latter frequently has ischemic and systemic manifestations as well.

O   **How does one diagnose carotid artery disease?**

Carotid bruits by physical exam. Duplex scanning provides both anatomic and hemodynamic information and may be the imaging study of choice. Arteriography, while excellent, does carry a significant stroke rate associated with the procedure (about 1 to 1.2 percent).

O   **How does one treat symptomatic carotid artery disease?**

In general, in patients with grater than 70% stenosis, surgery plus medical therapy in superior to medical therapy alone.

O   **List the causes of recurrent venous thrombosis.**

There are multiple etiologies, but may include idiopathic, Buerger's disease, ulcerative colitis connective tissue disease, oral contraceptive use, or neoplasm. Coagulation disorders are also part of the differential diagnosis.

O   **What are the congenital cardiovascular diseases associated with aortic dissection?**

Bicuspid aortic valve and coarctation of the aorta predispose to aorta dissection. Dissection has also been reported in Noonan syndrome and Turner's syndrome. Cystic degeneration is common to all these reports.

O   **What is the most common pathological feature predisposing to aortic dissection?**

Degeneration of the tunica media is considered a pre-requisite for development of aortic dissection. Pathologically this consists of deterioration of the collagen and elastic tissue, usually with cystic changes (Cystic Medial Necrosis).

O   **What is the most common cause of cystic medical necrosis?**

Cystic medial necrosis is most often the result of chronic stress to the aortic wall, such as occurs with long standing hypertension. Thus, hypertension is perhaps the single most important physiologic derangement leading to aortic dissection, occurring in a proximately 80% of patients. While medial degeneration is a normal part of the aging process, these changes are qualitatively and quantitatively greater in patients with aortic dissection.

O   **Which hereditary disorders are associated with aortic dissection?**

Marfan's disease and Ehlers-Danlos syndrome.

O   **What is the most common presenting symptoms of aortic dissection?**

Severe pain. The symptom is found in over 90% of patients. This pain is typically abrupt at onset, and often as severe at onset as it will ever get. Another feature of this symptom is the tendency to migrate from its origin and follow the physical path of the dissection.

O   **What are the other typical symptoms of aortic dissection?**

Diaphoresis, nausea, vomiting, apprehension and faintness.

O   **What is the most common reason for painless aortic dissection?**

Painless dissection usually results from loss of consciousness as a result of the dissection, leaving the patient unable to perceive pain (e.g. dissection of a carotid or vertebral artery). Painless dissection has been reported, however, in patients not presenting with loss of consciousness.

O   **When diagnosing pericardial effusion, how much fluid must be present in the pericardial sac for visualization on an cardiac echocardiography and by x-ray?**

At least 15 ml for an echocardiography and 250 ml for an x-ray.

O   **What will be the appearance of a pericardial effusion on an x-ray?**

A water-bottle silhouette.

O   **At what volume does pericardial effusion affect the intrapericardial pressure?**

80 to 200 ml. However, the rate of accumulation is more important than the amount of accumulation. If accumulated slowly, the pericardium can tolerate up to 2000 ml of fluid.

O   **What is the most common cause of pericardial effusions today?**

Malignant disease.

O   **What are the clinical and hemodynamic differences between constrictive pericarditis and restrictive cardiomyopathy?**

	Constrictive pericarditis	Restrictive cardiomyopathy
S 3 gallop	Absent	May be present

Pericardial knock	May be present	Absent
Palpable systolic apical impulse	Absent	May be present
Pericardial calcification	Present in 50%	Absent
Pulsus paradoxus	May be present	May be present
Equal RV and LV diastolic pressures	Usually present	LV>RV by more than 5 mm Hg
Rate of LV filling	80% in first half of diastole	40% in first half of diastole
PEP/LVET	Av. 0.31	Av. 0.48 (congestive failure)
CAT scan, echo, MRI	Thickened pericardium	Normal pericardium

○ **What is the hallmark of effusive-constrictive pericarditis?**

Continued elevation of the right atrial pressure after the aspiration of pericardial fluid and restoration of intrapericardial pressure to zero.

○ **What is the most common cause of fungal pericarditis?**

Histoplasmosis.

○ **What are the clinical and hemodynamic features of cardiac tamponade, subacute constrictive pericarditis and chronic "rigid" constrictive pericarditis?**

	Cardiac Tamponade	Subacute constriction	Chronic "rigid" constriction
Duration of symptoms	Hours to days	Weeks to months	Months to years
Chest pain, friction rub	Usual	Recent past	Remote
Pulsus paradoxus	Prominent	Usually prominent	Slight or absent
Kussmaul's sign	Absent	Usually absent	Often present
Early diastolic knock	Absent	Usually absent	Often present
Heart size on chest x-ray	Usually enlarged	Usually enlarged	Usually normal
Pericardial calcification	Absent	Rare	Often present
Abnormal P waves or atrial fibrillation	Absent	Absent	Often present
Venous (right atrial) waveform	X or Xy	Xy or XY	XY or xY
Pericardial effusion	Always present	Often present	Absent

X and Y = prominent x and y descents, respectively. x and y = inconspicuous x and descents.

CONGENITAL HEART DISEASE

O   **What is the most common cardiac malformation at birth?**

Ventricular septal defect.

O   **What is the most common cause of cardiac chest pain in a patient with congenital heart disease?**

Anomalous pulmonary origin of a coronary artery.

O   **What is the most reliable respiratory characteristics of congentital cyanotic cardiac disease?**

Tachypnea and increased depth of respiration in the presence of cyanosis, without respiratory distress, that does not respond to 100% oxygen, suggesting a right-to-left shunt.

O   **What is the most common atrial septal defect seen and what does it involve anatomically?**

Ostium secundum type, most often involving the fossa ovalis. It is usually mid-septal.

O   **What other cardiac abnormality is most commonly associated with atrial septal defect?**

Mitral valve prolapse, found in 10-20% of patients with ostium secundum atrial setpal defect.

O   **What are the most notable cardiac auscultatory findings in children with atrial septal defects?**

Normal or split first heart sound, accentuation of the tricuspid valve closure sound, a midsystolic pulmonary ejection murmur and a wide, fixed split second heart sound.

O   **What is the typical CXR findings of a patient with atrial septal defect?**

Enlargement of the right atrium and ventricle, dilated pulmonary artery and its branches, and increased pulmonary vascular markings.

O   **Sinus venosus atrial septal defect is associated with what other cardiac anomaly?**

Anomalous pulmonary venous drainage, although this may less commonly occur with secundum defects.

O   **What is the confirmatory test of choice for atrial septal defect?**

Echocardiography with color Doppler flow and contrast echocardiography.

O   **When should surgical repair be considered for patients with atrial septal defect and when is the optimal timing for such treatment?**

Surgical repair should be carried out in all patients with atrial septal defect who have evidence of a left-to-right shunt where there is a pulmonary-to-systemic flow ratio equal to or greater than 1.5 : 1.0 determined by cardiac catheterization. The cardiac catheterization should ideally be carried out in patients between 2 and 4 years of age. Surgical therapy should not be carried out in patients with small defects and trivial left-to-right shunts (less than 1.5 : 1.0) or in patients with severe pulmonary hypertension without a significant left-to-right shunt.

○   **What non-cardiac problem is most common in children with atrial septal defect?**

Respiratory infections. They must be treated promptly to avoid the unlikely, but devastating consequences of infective endocarditis.

○   **What is the most common clinical symptom of patients with atrial septal defect, regardless of age?**

Exertional dyspnea and fatigue.

○   **What percentage of congenital heart defects do AV septal defects (also known as endocardial cushion defects and AV canal defects) account for?**

4-5%.

○   **What other congenital abnormalities are associated with AV septal defects?**

Asplenia or polysplenia syndromes, Down's syndrome, polydactyly, and Ellis-van Creveld syndrome of ectodermal dysplasia.

○   **What is the most common ECG finding in ostium secundum atrial septal defect?**

Right axis deviation, right ventricular hypertrophy and rSR in the right precordial leads with a normal QRS duration.

○   **What ECG abnormality suggests a sinus venosus defect rather than an ostium secundum defect?**

A negative P wave in lead III.

○   **Which valve is most often involved ion an ostium primum atrial septal defect?**

The mitral valve anterior leaflets are often displaced and commonly cleft, and the tricuspid valve is not commonly involved.

○   **What is the most common ECG findings in ostium primum atrial septal defect?**

Left anterior fascicular block, left axis deviation, prolongation of the P-R interval and counterclockwise rotation of the QRS loop in the frontal plane.

○   **What are the echocardiographic features of an AV septal defect?**

RV and pulmonary artery dilatation, systolic anterior anterior ventricular septal motion, and dropout of the inferior portion of the interatrial septum.

○   **What other features, besides those of all AV septal defects, are found in complete AV septal defects?**

Ventricular septal defects in the posterior basal inlet portion of the ventricular septum and a common AV valve.

○   **How many leaflets does the common AV valve in complete AV septal defect have?**

Six.

○   **What other cardiovascular lesions are associated with complete AV septal defect (common AV canal) and how common are they?**

35% of patients with common AV canal have additional cardiovascular lesions, most commonly Tetralogy of Fallot, double-outlet right ventricle, transposition of the great vessels, and asplenia and polysplenia syndromes.

○   **What other congenital abnormality is most commonly associated with Type A complete AV septal defect?**

Down's syndrome.

○   **What are the most common clinical symptoms in infants with complete AV septal defects?**

Heart failure, frequent respiratory infections and poor weight gain, usually occurring before 1 year of age.

○   **What are the most common physical findings in patients with complete AVA septal defects?**

Right ventricular precordial heave, a wide and fixed split second heart sound, a systolic ejection murmur heard best at the right sternal border in the 4th intercostal space, a mid-diastolic tricuspid flow rumble, and may include a holosystolic lower left sternal border murmur of an interventricular communication and/or the decrescendo, holosystolic apical murmur of mitral regurgitation.

○   **What are the ECG findings characteristic of complete AV canal defects?**

They resemble those of ostium primum AV septal defect, i.e., left anterior fascicular block, left axis deviation, prolongation of the P-R interval and counterclockwise rotation of the QRS loop in the frontal plane.

○   **What are the findings on cardiac catheterization of complete AV canal defects?**

Diagnosis is reliably established by selective LV angiography showing absence of the AV septum, deficiency of the inlet portion of the ventricular septum, elongation of the LV outflow tract in relation to the inflow tract, elevation and displacement of the aortic valve, marked elevation of pulmonary arterial pressure, and "gooseneck" deformity of the aorta seen angiographically in diastole.

○   **What is the management goal in patients with complete AV canal defects?**

Control of cardiac decompensation, followed by surgical repair, preferrably by the age of 6 months so as to avoid or minimize obstructive pulmonary vascular disease.

○   **Where do the most common ventricular septal defects occur in the septum?**

Most commonly in the region of the membranous septum.

○   **What are the three different types of ventricular septal defects?**

Perimembranous, muscular, and subpulmonary. Perimembranous are the most common.

○   **What is the best test to identify the type and severity of ventricular septal defect?**

2-D and Doppler echocardiography.

○   **What percentage of ventricular septal defects spontaneously close?**

45% completely close by age 3, another 15% completely close by age 15. Partial, rather than complete, closure is common in patients with both large and small ventricular septal defects. Even 7% of patients with large VSD's and early CHF will experience closure of their VSD.

○ **What is the most common physical finding in a patient with a large VSD?**

Holosystolic murmur best heard at the lower left sternal border with a thrill and a low-pitched diastolic rumble at the apex.

○ **What is the most important prognostic factor in the pre-operative evaluation of patients with large VSD's?**

The degree of elevated pulmonary vascular resistance. If the pre-operative pulmonary vascular resistance is one-third that of the systemic circulation or less, then the progression of pulmonary hypertension is unusual and the prognosis is good. However, if the pulmonary vascular resistance pre-operatively is moderately or severely elevated, then the prognosis is less favorable and progression of pulmonary hypertension is likely post-operatively.

○ **What is the most common cardiac complication of ventricular septal defect and how common is it?**

Aortic regurgitation is well-described and occurs in about 5% of patients, usually noted after age 5. It is more common in Japan than in the United States or Europe.

○ **Is it necessary to restrict the activities of children with isolated ventricular septal defect?**

Usually not. Antibiotic prophylaxis is indicated for dental procedures and minor surgery as infective endocarditis is always a threat. Respiratory infections must be promptly evaluated and treated and children with VSD's should be checked once or twice per year to detect changes in the clinical picture that suggest the development of pulmonary vascular obliterative changes. Surgery should be electively planned only when the shunt is large enough (> 2.0 : 1 pulmonary-systemic flow ratios).

○ **What is the most common post-operative complication following surgical repair of VSD?**

Complete AV block.

○ **What is the therapy for patients with Eisenmenger's right to left shunt in patients with VSD?**

There is little to offer this group of patients other than supportive care and maximal medical therapy to slow the progression of hemodynamic deterioration.

○ **What are the features of Tetralogy of Fallot?**

1. Ventricular septal defect
2. Obstruction of the right ventricular outflow tract
3. Overriding of the aorta
4. Right ventricular hypertrophy

○ **What is the incidence of Tetralogy of Fallot in relationship to all forms of congenital heart disease?**

The overall incidence of this anomaly approaches 10% of all forms of congenital heart disease, and it is the most common cardiac malformation responsible for cyanosis after 1 year of age.

○ **Associated cardiac anomalies exist in what percentage of patients with Tetralogy of Fallot?**

40%. They include patent ductus arteriosus, multiple (usually muscular) ventricular septal defects, and complete AV septal defects. Coronary artery and pulmonary artery anomalies are common and unilateral absence of a pulmonary artery may be found in a small number of patients.

O   **What is the treatment of patients with Tetralogy of Fallot?**

Total surgical correction at the earliest possible time. The anatomy of the right ventricular outflow tract and the size of the pulmonary arteries, rather than the age or size of the infant or child, are the most important factors in assessing candidacy for primary repair. Marked hypoplasia of the pulmonary arteries demands a palliative operation designed to increase pulmonary blood flow. Primary repair in those patients can then be carried out later in childhood.

O   **What are some of the systemic conditions that may exist in patients with Tetralogy of Fallot?**

Polycythemia, iron deficiency anemia, infective endocarditis, paradoxical embolism, cerebrovascular accidents, coagulation disorders and cerebral abscess.

O   **What is Ebstein's anomaly?**

This malformation is characterized by a downward displacement of the tricuspid valve into the right ventricle due to anomalous attachment of the tricuspid leaflets. Tricuspid valve tissue is dysplastic and a variable portion of the septal and inferior cusps adhere to the right ventricular wall some distance away from the AV junction.
Thus, a portion of the right ventricle lies between the AV ring and the origin of the valve and is "atrialized". A small, often dysfunctional right ventricular chamber exists.

O   **What other congenital abnormalities are associated with Ebstein's anomaly?**

The most common and important associated defect is pulmonary stenosis or atresia. Patent foramen ovale or an ostium secundum atrial septal defect occur in over half the cases. Ebstein's anomaly is commonly associated with congenitally corrected transposition of the great vessels.

O   **What are the most common manifestations in Ebstein's anomaly?**

In infancy, cyanosis is the most common, along with a cardiac murmur and severe congestive heart failure. Beyond infancy, the onset of symptoms is insidious and the most common symptoms are exertional dyspnea, fatigue and cyanosis. About 25% of patients suffer episodes of paroxysmal atrial tachycardia.

O   **What are the auscultatory findings in patients with Ebstein's anomaly?**

A holosystolic murmur of tricuspid regurgitation, often with a thrill, wide splitting of the first and second heart sounds and a prominent S3 or S4, producing a characteristic rhythmic auscultatory cadence with a triple, quadruple or quintuple combination of sounds.

O   **What is the management of patients with Ebstein's anomaly?**

In symptomatic infants, the surgical approach is similar to patients with tricuspid atresia, creating a systemic pulmonary shunt, and at a later age, the Fontan approach. In older patients, significant benefit has resulted from reconstruction of the tricuspid valve, closure of the atrial septal defect, plication of the free wall of the right ventricle, posterior tricuspid annuloplasty and a reduction in right atrial size.
Those patients with life-threatening pre-excitation syndrome, ablation of accessory pathways via catheter or surgery are undertaken. All patients with symtomatic Ebstein's anomaly or those asymptomatic patients with significant cardiac enlargement should have surgery.

O   **What type of intracardiac shunt is most frequently associated with pulmonary hypertension?**

A ventricular septal defect (VSD).

O   **What radiographic finding is associated with transposition of the great vessels?**

An egg-shaped heart.

O   **What are the pathophysiologic consequences of a left-to-right intracardiac shunt?**

Diastolic overloading, cardiac dilatation and ventricular enlargement.

O   **PDA arises from which aortic arch?**

The left sixth arch.

O   **What is the hallmark of PDA?**

A continuous machinery murmur associated with a widened pulse pressure.

O   **What are the chest x-ray findings associated with PDA?**

Left ventricular hypertrophy (LVH), increased vascular markings and an enlarged pulmonary conus.
O   **What is the definitive diagnostic test for PDA?**

Aortography.

O   **What is the treatment of choice for premature infants with PDA?**

Indomethacin.

O   **What are the four types of VSD?**

Perimembranous, supracristal, atrioventricular canal and muscular.

O   **PDA accounts for what percentage of congenital heart defects?**

15%.

O   **What are the four types of total anomalous pulmonary venous drainage?**

Supracardiac, intracardiac, infracardiac and mixed.

O   **What is the classic radiographic finding associated with coarctation of the aorta?**

Rib-notching.

O   **T/F: ECG accurately determines the severity of obstruction in patients with pulmonic stenosis.**

True.

O   **Right atrial enlargement is associated with which congenital heart defects?**

Ebstein's malformation, ASD and pulmonic stenosis.

○   **What is the hallmark of congestive heart failure (CHF) in children?**

Hepatic enlargement.

○   **What is the etiology of transposition of the great vessels?**

Abnormal development of the primitive bulbus cordis.

○   **What congenital heart defects result in obstructive lesions and increased ventricular work?**

Pulmonic stenosis, aortic stenosis and coarctation of the aorta.

○   **What is the appropriate therapy for a newborn with IHSS?**

Continuous infusion of prostaglandin E1 (PGE1), low FIO2 and a Norwood repair.

○   **When do intracardiac shunts become physiologically important?**

When the pulmonary blood flow exceeds 1.5 to 2 times the systemic flow.

○   **What concomitant cardiac defect is required for survival for patients with total anomalous pulmonary venous drainage?**

A patent ASD.

○   **What is the etiology of the gracile habitus in children with a PDA or ASD?**

The shunt causes an increased blood flow through the pulmonary vasculature and decreased flow through the systemic vasculature, resulting in retardation of normal growth and development.

○   **T/F: Squatting can increase systemic vascular resistance (SVR) and, thus, decrease right-to-left shunting.**

True.

○   **What are cyanotic spells?**

Periodic episodes of unconsciousness related to cerebral hypoxia.

○   **What radiologic finding is associated with Tetralogy of Fallot?**

A sabot-shaped heart.

○   **What auscultatory finding is associated with PDA?**

A widely split and "fixed" S2.

○   **Which congenital heart defects are associated with congenital aortic stenosis?**

PDA, VSD, coarctation of the aorta and mitral valve defects.

○   **An 8 year-old male is brought to the ER by his mother who states he has been having chest pain. Physical exam reveals a systolic ejection murmur and a precordial thrill. Chest x-ray is normal. What is the treatment of choice?**

Aortic valve replacement.

O   **What are the characteristics of the absent pulmonary valve variant of Tetralogy of Fallot?**

VSD, pulmonary stenosis, tracheobronchial malacia and stenosis.

O   **T/F: Isoproterenol is the appropriate treatment for intractable "tet spells" (hypercyanotic spell of Tetralogy of Fallot).**

False.

O   **T/F: The Waterson shunt is an appropriate option for a newborn with severe cyanosis due to Tetralogy of Fallot.**

True.

O   **What ECG findings differentiate an ostium primum from an ostium secundum ASD?**

Left axis deviation and counterclockwise rotation of the vectorgram is associated with an ostium primum defect and right axis deviation and a right bundle branch block pattern are associated with an ostium secundum defect.

O   **What is the etiology of the typical heart murmur seen in patients with an ASD?**

Flow across the pulmonic valve.

O   **What is involved in the repair of an AV canal defect?**

Placing a patch to close the VSD, another patch to close the atrial septal defect and division and resuspension of the common AV valve into a left sided (corresponding to the mitral valve) and right sided (corresponding to the tricuspid valve) component.

O   **A 6 month-old with a VSD undergoes cardiac catheterization with the following findings:**

Site	Oxygen saturation	Pressure (mm Hg)
Superior vena cava	65%	5
Right atrium	66%	5
Right ventricle	75%	70/5
Pulmonary artery	90%	65/20
Left atrium	98%	7
Left ventricle	98%	75/7
Aorta	98%	75/40

What is the diagnosis?

Transposition of the great vessels.

O   **At what age should the arterial switch procedure be performed for patients with transposition of the great vessels?**

Usually at 1 to 2 weeks of age

What is the degree of left to right shunt?

4:1. $(SaO_2 - SvO_2) / (SpvO_2 - SpaO_2)$, where SaO_2 is the systemic arterial oxygen saturation (aorta), SvO_2 is the mixed venous oxygen saturation (superior vena cava), $SpvO_2$ is the oxygen saturation in the pulmonary veins (left atrium) and $SpaO_2$ is the oxygen saturation in the pulmonary artery.

O   A 4 day-old infant presents with shock and severe acidosis. Echocardiogram demonstrates an interrupted aortic arch, type B. What is the next step in management?

Continuous infusion of prostaglandin E1.

O   What disorder is likely to accompany the patient in the question above?

DiGeorge syndrome (thymic aplasia).

O   T/F: Aortic dissection is a potential long term complication of the Fontan procedure.

False.

O   A 9 month-old child has progressive cyanosis but is otherwise asymptomatic. Echocardiogram demonstrates Tetralogy of Fallot. Complete repair is contemplated and cardiac catheterization is proposed. What is the most important information to be obtained from the catheterization?

The coronary artery anatomy.

O   A 6 month-old presents with sweating and irritability while feeding. Chest x-ray demonstrates a markedly enlarged cardiac silhouette and echocardiogram reveals a dilated, poorly contractile left ventricle with moderate to severe mitral regurgitation. What is the most likely diagnosis?

Anomalous origin of the left coronary artery from the pulmonary artery.

O   T/F: Anomalous left coronary artery from the pulmonary artery is best treated by reimplantation of the coronary artery into the aorta.

True.

O   What congenital heart lesion is the most common cause of cyanosis presenting in the newborn period?

Transposition of the great vessels.

O   What complications are associated with surgical repair of coarctation of the aorta?

Paraplegia and postoperative hypertension.

O   An 8 year-old child presents with cyanosis but is otherwise asymptomatic. Cardiac catheterization reveals the following:

Site	Oxygen saturation	Pressure (mm Hg)
Superior vena cava	61%	5
Right atrium	62%	5
Right ventricle	4%	100/5
Pulmonary artery	67%	100/60
Left atrium	98%	8
Left ventricle	89%	100/8
Aorta	82%	100/70

What is the most likely diagnosis?

VSD with high pulmonary vascular resistance (Eisenmenger's syndrome).

❍   **T/F: Coarctation of the aorta is associated with total anomalous pulmonary venous drainage.**

False.

❍   **What percentage of adults have a patent foramen ovale?**

10 to 20%.

❍   **Why is a paradoxical embolus able to cause septic end-organ disease?**

An infected venous thrombus can enter the arterial circulation via a right-to-left intracardiac shunt and be sent distal to affect end-organs.

❍   **What is the normal shunt fraction?**

10%.

❍   **What is the pathophysiology of Eisenmenger's syndrome?**

Pulmonary vascular resistance (PVR) increasing to levels greater than systemic vascular resistance (SVR) resulting in reversal of the original left-to-right shunt and cyanosis.

❍   **What is the main contraindication to surgical closure of a PDA?**

Cyanosis.

❍   **What is the most frequently used palliative procedure for patients with Tetralogy of Fallot?**

A subclavian artery-to-pulmonary artery (Blalock-Taussig) shunt.

❍   **What is the treatment of choice for patients with transposition of the great vessels?**

The arterial switch procedure.

❍   **What ECG findings are diagnostic for tricuspid atresia?**

Left ventricular hypertrophy (LVH) and left axis deviation.

❍   **Which congenital heart defect is associated with the presence of an abnormal chamber superior and posterior to the left atrium?**

Cor triatriatum.

❍   **What is the etiology of an aortopulmonary window?**

Abnormal separation of the primitive truncus arteriosus into the aorta and pulmonary artery.

❍   **Which cardiac valve is most frequently affected in patients with truncus arteriosus?**

The tricuspid valve.

❍   **What percentage of premature infants have successful closure of a PDA with indomethacin?**

50%.

O   **What are the relative contraindications to the use of indomethacin for neonates with PDA?**

Intracranial hemorrhage, nephritis and enterocolitis.

O   **What is the most common etiology of congenital aortic stenosis?**

Fusion of the commissure between the right and left coronary cusps.

O   **What indicates severe disease in previously asymptomatic congenital aortic stenosis?**

Valvular calcifications.

O   **What is the prognosis for patients with a complete atrioventricular canal?**

Cardiac enlargement and severe cardiac failure in the first few years of life with a mortality rate of 5 to 15%.

O   **What concomitant cardiac defect is required for survival for patients with total anomalous pulmonary venous drainage?**

A patent atrial septal defect (ASD).

O   **T/F: Partial anomalous pulmonary venous drainage usually arises from the right lung.**

True.

O   **Where do left anomalous pulmonary veins usually enter the systemic circulation?**

Through a persistent left subclavian vein.

O   **What is the palliative treatment for infants with total anomalous venous drainage until definitive surgical correction can be performed?**

Balloon septoplasty.

O   **What is the scimitar syndrome?**

The radiographic appearance created by the shadow of an anomalous right pulmonary vein arising parallel to the right border of the heart and entering the inferior vena cava (IVC) or right atrium.

O   **T/F: Congestive heart failure (CHF) usually develops in children with a right-to-left intracardiac shunt.**

False.

O   **What factors affect the degree of cyanosis in patients with a right-to-left intracardiac shunt?**

The severity of anoxia and the concentration of blood hemoglobin.

O   **Left atrial enlargement is associated with which congenital heart defects?**

Mitral insufficiency, patent ductus arteriosus (PDA) and VSD.

O   **What auscultatory finding is associated with PDA?**

A widely split and "fixed" S2.

○   **Which congenital heart defects are associated with congenital aortic stenosis?**

PDA, VSD, coarctation of the aorta and mitral valve defects.

○   **T/F: ECG accurately determines the severity of obstruction in patients with pulmonic stenosis.**

True.

○   **What is the most common form of a univentricular heart (UVH)?**

A double-inlet right ventricle.

○   **What is the mortality rate for infants with uncorrected transposition of the great vessels?**

90%.

○   **What congenital heart lesions result in a continuous (systolic and diastolic) murmur.**

PDA, aortopulmonary window and coronary arteriovenous fistula.

○   **What is the etiology of an AV canal defect?**

Underdevelopment of the endocardial cushions, leaving a large inlet VSD, a large primum atrial septal defect and a common AV valve separating the atria from the ventricles.

○   **A 12-hour-old newborn presents with respiratory distress, cyanosis and diffuse interstitial edema on chest x-ray. An echocardiogram demonstrates total anomalous pulmonary venous return. What is the most appropriate next step in treatment?**

Total anomalous pulmonary venous drainage.

○   **What is the most common late complication of the arterial switch procedure?**

Supravalvular pulmonic stenosis.

○   **Where do aneurysms of the right coronary sinus of Valsalva usually rupture?**

Into the right ventricle.

○   **What are the clinical characteristics of Ebstein's anomaly?**

Varying degrees of deformity of the tricuspid valve with associated obstruction to egress of blood from the right ventricle, severe tricuspid regurgitation and an enlarged cardiac silhouette seen on chest x-ray.

CARDIAC PHARMACOLOGY

O   **Calcium use is de-emphasized but is still indicated for which situations?**

Hyperkalemia, hypocalcemia and calcium channel blocker toxicity.

O   **Why is bretylium a second line pharmacologic treatment for ventricular ectopy after lidocaine?**

Bretylium is associated with hypotension and increased myocardial oxygen consumption, both undesirable effects in the setting of ischemic heart disease.

O   **How do inotropic agents increase myocardial contractility?**

By increasing intracellular calcium concentration and availability.

O   **What is the most common side effect of esmolol, labetalol, and bretylium?**

Hypotension.

O   **What side effect can occur with a rapid infusion of procainamide?**

Hypotension. Other side effects include QRS/QT prolongation, ventricular fibrillation, and Torsade de pointes.

O   **What are some adverse drug effects of lidocaine?**

Drowsiness, nausea, vertigo, confusion, ataxia, tinnitus, muscle twitching, respiratory depression, and psychosis.

O   **Which do nitrates affect, preload or afterload?**

Predominantly preload.

O   **Which does hydralazine affect, preload or afterload?**

Predominantly afterload.

O   **Do prazosin, captopril, and nifedipine affect afterload?**

Yes.

O   **When is dobutamine used in CHF?**

When heart failure is not accompanied with severe hypotension. Dobutamine is a potent inotrope with some vasodilation activity.

O   **When is dopamine selected in CHF?**

When a patient is in shock. Dopamine is a vasoconstrictor and a positive inotrope.

○ **Lovastatin (Mevacor) and niacin are used to treat hyperlipoproteinemia. Both of these drugs lower triglycerides and LDL. Which one raises HDL?**

Only niacin. Lovastatin has little affect on HDL. However, because niacin often produces significant side effects, such as gastritis, reactivation of peptic ulcers, gout, hyperglycemia, cutaneous flushing, and scaling skin, Lovastatin remains the first-line drug of choice.

○ **While taking your boards, why might you become severely annoyed if seated next to a person on ACE inhibitors?**

ACE inhibitors produce a cough in 5-15% of patients.

○ **What are the most common side effects of beta-blockers?**

Fatigue will occur early in treatment, followed later by depression. Impotence is also commonly reported.

○ **What are the side effects of thiazide diuretics?**

Hyperglycemia, hyperlipidemia, hyperuricemia, hypokalemia, hypomagnesemia, and hyponatremia.

○ **What is the agent of choice in diabetic patients with hypertension?**

ACE inhibitors.

○ **What drugs have been shown to regress LV hypertrophy and reduce LV mass?**

Beta-blockers, verapamil, alpha-methyldopa (Aldomet), ACE inhibitors, and thiazide diuretics.

○ **Which agent is more likely to cause bradycardia, verapamil or diltiazem?**

Diltiazem. Diltiazem blocks conduction through both the SA and AV node, whereas verapamil blocks only the AV node.

○ **Which drugs can increase serum digoxin levels?**

Quinidine, procainamide, verapamil, and amiodarone.

○ **What is the most frequent side effect of verapamil?**

Constipation.

○ **What are the most frequent side effects of nifedipine?**

Lower extremity edema, dizziness, and headache.

○ **What pharmacologic agent should be avoided in a patient with paroxysmal atrial fibrillation who is presently in sinus rhythm?**

Dihydropyridine calcium channel blockers, such as nifedipine. They predispose patients to relapse back into atrial fibrillation.

○ **What medications, used to maintain sinus rhythm in a patient recently cardioverted from atrial fibrillation, should be avoided in patients with stress-test proven myocardial ischemia?**

Class 1C antiarrhythmics, such as flecainide and propafenone and class 1A agents, such as quinidine and procainamide. They can lead to lethal proarrhythmia in patients with active myocardial ischemia. Amiodarone, an agent that has anti-ischemic properties, is the preferred agent.

O   **What antihypertensive agents are preferred agents to use in a 63 year-old obese, African-American male?**

Diuretics and/or ACE inhibitors.

O   **Which drugs should be administered to lower the BP in a patient with thoracic aortic dissection?**

Sodium nitroprusside, propranolol, esmolol or labetalol.

O   **You administer 6 mg adenosine through a peripheral IV to break an SVT. Nothing happens! Now what?**

Adenosine's half-life is 10 seconds, and it can be "lost" in the periphery. Follow its administration with a rapid saline flush. Consider an additional 12 mg bolus five minutes later if 6 mg doesn't work.

O   **Immediately after a "chemical stress test" an elderly woman with peripheral vascular disease develops SVT. 6 mg of adenosine is administered. Now the patient is asystolic. What happened?**

Dipyridamole, the likely chemical used in the stress test above, potentiates the effects of adenosine. In such patients, smaller doses of adenosine should be used.

O   **You administer 6 mg of adenosine to a young patient with SVT. He experiences the sudden onset of sever chest pain and shortness of breath. What happened?**

Flushing, palpitations, chest pain and shortness of breath are common, and short-lived, effects of adenosine administration.

O   **A patient followed for severe chronic obstructive pulmonary disease has an SVT that shows no response to adenosine. Why?**

This patient may be on a methylxanthine preparation. Methylxanthines antagonize the effects of adenosine.

O   **What is the likely response of atrial tachycardia to vagal maneuvers or adenosine?**

A practical way of classifying SVT is by response to adenosine. In junctional (AV node-dependent) tachycardias, such as AV node reentry or AV reentry (a bypass track is part of the circuit), the AV node is an essential part of the tachycardia mechanism: if conduction through the AV node is blocked, the tachycardia will terminate. In atrial (AV node-independent) tachycardias, of which sinus tachycardia, sinus node reentry tachycardia, atrial tachycardia, and atrial fibrillation and flutter are examples, the nidus of the arrhythmia is within the atria and is not affected by conduction through the AV node. Therefore, in atrial tachycardia, ventricular conduction will be blocked, but atrial activity will continue.

O   **What agents should never be administered in the above clinical setting?**

Digoxin or verapamil.

O   **An ICU patient develops SVT that you suspect is due to cyclic antidepressant toxicity. What antiarrhythmic agents should not be used?**

Type 1A (i.e., quinidine and procainamide) and type 1C (i.e., flecainide) agents have similar cardiotoxic and anticholinergic effects as cyclic antidepressants. Bretylium may worsen toxicity-related hypotension.

○   **Fifteen minutes after receiving thrombolysis for acute MI, your patient develops worsening chest pain and anterior ST elevations, and a wide-complex rhythm at 100 bpm. The rhythm soon and the patient's pain and ST segment elevation dramatically improve. What happened?**

Accelerated idioventricular rhythm (AIVR) or "slow VT" often accompanies clinical signs and symptoms of reperfusion, and is often referred to as a "reperfusion arrhythmia". Patients should be carefully observed but usually no specific treatment is necessary for this rhythm.

○   **A 45 year-old smoker presents with symptoms of palpitations and is found to be in a regular, wide complex tachycardia at a rate of 170 bpm. He is reclining comfortably on a stretcher while you interview him (and sweat). What can you safely assume about the etiology of his tachycardia?**

Assume only one thing: This is ventricular tachycardia! It is VT! Almost any regular wide-complex tachycardia in an adult should be assumed to be VT until proved otherwise. "Hemodynamic stability" is a useless criterion for assuming SVT.

○   **What is the most important question you should ask the above patient about his past medical history?**

If he had an MI. A past history of MI raises the likelihood of a wide complex tachycardia being ventricular tachycardia to greater than 90%. Age greater than 65 and past VT also raise the ante.

○   **What is the differential diagnosis of a regular, wide-complex tachycardia?**

Ventricular tachycardia, supraventricular tachycardia with aberrancy, or supraventricular tachycardia with antegrade conduction down an accessory pathway (antidromic tachycardia).

○   **What is aberrant conduction?**

During normal antegrade AV conduction, there is delay or block of conduction in the His-Purkinje system. Rate-dependent aberrancy, as might be seen at the onset of a rapid SVT, is in the differential of wide-complex tachycardia, as noted above, and can be confused with VT.

○   **How can a previous 12 lead ECG help distinguish between VT and SVT with aberrancy?**

If wide complex tachycardia has the same bundle branch morphology as a previous ECG in sinus rhythm, it is likely to be SVT with aberrancy. Conversely, if the wide complex pattern is different from that noted in sinus rhythm, then the wide complex tachycardia is most likely VT.

○   **How can isolated ectopic complexes help distinguish between VT and SVT with aberrancy?**

Beats that look like PVC's on ECG's or rhythm strips and that have the same morphology (i.e., in the same lead) during a wide complex tachycardia suggest VT as the etiology of the sustained tachycardia.

○   **How are tachycardia rate and slight irregularity of tachycardia cycle length useful in distinguishing VT from SVT with aberrancy?**

They are not. A very irregular wide complex tachycardia suggests atrial fibrillation with conduction over an accessory pathway, especially at very rapid rates.

○   **Name important physical exam findings in VT.**

The classical teaching is that A-V dissociation is present in VT (but see below!). Since filling of the LV will vary depending on the (dissociated) relationship of the atria and ventricles, the intensity of S1 will vary. With dissociation, the atria should be contracting against closed AV valves now and again: the presence of "cannon" A waves in the neck veins strongly suggests VT. Since S1 will vary, so will LV ejection on a beat-to-beat basis: Varying intensity of the peripheral pulse or intermittent Korotkoff sounds may be present.

○ What percentage of VT does not exhibit AV dissociation?

Up to 25% of patients have intact VA conduction (retrograde conduction) during VT. Obviously they will not exhibit cannon A waves. It is possible for AV dissociation to occur in SVT, but this is a rare phenomenon.

○ What is the most common tachycardia associated with pulmonary embolism?

Sinus tachycardia. This old saw works backwards too: unexplained tachycardia in a patient who doesn't look right and is making you nervous should make you think of pulmonary embolism.

○ During attempted cardioversion of atrial flutter with procainamide, you note that the ventricular rate, 150 bpm prior to infusion, has accelerated to 200. What happened?

You did not "block down" the AV node with a beta blocker, a calcium channel blocker, or digoxin. Class 1A agents (quinidine, procainamide and disopyramide) have vagolytic properties and slow the rate of flutter, both of which can lead to an increase in the flutter rate.

○ What agent has clearly emerged as the first-choice drug in the restoration of sinus rhythm in new-onset atrial fibrillation?

There is no consensus. Stay tuned; this is a controversial topic.

○ What is ibutilide? What might it effectively treat? What important caveats are there to its use?

Ibutilide is a new Class III antiarrhythmic agent. In a recent placebo-controlled, dose-ranging study, ibutilide was found to have a greater than 40% success rate in converting new-onset atrial fibrillation to sinus rhythm at highest doses, and to do so in a mean time of only 19 minutes. However, 3.6% of patients developed polymorphic VT, and 1% required immediate cardioversion. Patients administered ibutilide require at least 4 hours of monitoring after infusion.

○ A 75 year-old man with a history of systolic heart failure was recently admitted for an episode of paroxysmal atrial fibrillation. He returns to the hospital confused, with a large right flank hematoma. He is in sinus rhythm on EKG. He cannot give you a history. However, he is clutching a bottle of amiodarone in his hand. Describe a likely scenario.

He was receiving appropriate therapy for heart failure/rate control with digoxin, and was placed on warfarin to prevent stroke in the setting of paroxysmal atrial fibrillation. The amiodarone was likely prescribed to maintain sinus rhythm. However, amiodarone increases digoxin levels and inhibits warfarin metabolism; it is likely that the dosages of the latter two drugs were not reduced – explaining the confusion (likely fall) and severe hematoma.

○ A 55 year-old man with hypertension presents with shortness of breath and atrial fibrillation of uncertain duration. He receives rate control and IV heparin. A transesophageal echocardiogram reveals no left atrial appendage thrombus. He is subsequently successfully cardioverted to sinus rhythm and discharged on no medications. Three days later he presents with a CVA. Why?

Although there may be no clot present at the time of cardioversion, atria may be "stunned" from prolonged fibrillation and need time for mechanical recovery. Thus, clot can form even when the patient is in sinus rhythm. For this reason, anticoagulation is usually maintained for several weeks after cardioversion.

❍   **What is the role of digoxin in converting patients in atrial fibrillation to sinus rhythm?**

There is none.

❍   **What is the treatment for verapamil-induced hypotension?**

Calcium gluconate 1 gram IV over several minutes.

❍   **A patient, who has a psychiatric history and is taking an MAO inhibitor, has consumed a 12-pack of beer with a meal of pickled herring and a nicely-aged cheese. He now complains of severe headache. Upon examination, his BP is elevated. A diagnosis of acute hypertension is made secondary to hyperstimulation of the adrenergic receptors. What is the treatment?**

An alpha and beta-adrenergic antagonist, such as labetalol.

❍   **What is the most common complication of nitroprusside?**

Hypotension. Thiocyanate toxicity, accompanied by blurred vision, tinnitus, change in mental status, muscle weakness, and seizures, is more prevalent in patients with renal failure or prolonged infusions. Cyanide toxicity is uncommon. However, this type of toxicity may occur with hepatic dysfunction, after prolonged infusions, and in rates greater than 10 mg/kg per minute.

❍   **What is the affect of a dopamine infusion greater than 5 ug/kg/min?**

Peripheral arterial vasoconstriction.

❍   **What are the end-points in procainamide loading infusion for patient with unstable VT?**

Hypotension, QRS widened more than 50% of pre-treatment width, arrhythmia suppression, or a total of 17 mg/kg.

❍   **Review the pharmacophysiologic effects of the vasodilators used in the treatment of congestive heart failure.**

Drug	Mechanism	Preload Reduction	Afterload Reduction
Renin-Angiotensin Antagonists			
Captopril	Inhibition of renal systemic	++	++
Enalapril	and tissue generation of	++	++
Quinapril	angiotensin II by ACE;	++	++
Lisinopril	decreased metabolism of	++	++
Ramipril	bradykinin	++	++
Fosinopril		++	++
Enalaprilat		++	++
Losartan	Blockade of angiotensin II	++	++
Candesartan	receptors (AT-1)	++	++
Nitrovasodilators			
Nitroglycerin	Nitric oxide donors	+++	+
Isosorbite Dinitrate	(Endothelial cell relaxing	+++	+
Isosorbide Mononitrate	factor-ERF)	+++	+
Nitroprusside		+++	+++

Direct Vasodilators

Hydralazine	Unclear	+	+++
Minoxidil	Increased potassium	+	+++
Diazoxide	channel conductance and other mechanisms	+	+++

Phosphodiesterase Inhibitors

Amrinone	Inhibition of type III cAMP	++	++
Milrinone	phosphodiesterase(s) and other mechanisms	++	++

Sympathomimetics

Dobutamine	Myocardial and vascular beta-adrenergic agonist	+	++
Dopamine	Selective renal arterial vasodilation		
Low dose (<3mcg/kg/min)		0	+/-
High dose(4-20 mcg/kg/min)		++	—

Calcium Channel Blockers

Nifedipine	Inhibition of L-type voltage-	+	+++
Amlodipine	sensitive calcium channels	+	+++
Felodipine		+	+++
Diltiazem	Same as above (use in predominantly diastolic heart failure)	+	+/++
Verapamil	Same as above (use only in diastolic heart failure)	+	+++

Sympatholytics

Prazosin	Alpha-1-adrenergic receptor	+++	+
Terazosin	antagonists	+++	+
Carvedilol	Combined alpha-1 and beta	+	++
Labetolol	adrenergic blockade	+	++

○ **What are the factors favoring deterioration of renal function when using ACE inhibitors in patients with congestive heart failure?**

1. Hyponatremia (serum Na less than 130
2. Prerenal azotemia
3. Mean arterial pressure less than 80 mm Hg
4. Co-administration of prostaglandin inhibitors
5. Presence of adrenergic dysfunction (e.g. diabetes mellitus)
6. Large doses of diuretics
7. Evidence of maximal neurohumoral activation

○ **What are the factors favoring improvement of renal function when using ACE inhibitors in patients with congestive heart failure?**

1. Normal serum sodium and maintenance of sodium balance
2. Mean arterial pressure greater than 80 mm Hg
3. Minimal neurohumoral activation
4. Intact counterregulatory mechanisms
5. Reduction in diuretic dosage

6.   Increase in sodium intake

HYPERTENSION

○ **Has the prevalence of hypertension increased, decreased or remained unchanged over the last 20 years in the United States?**

Increased, because the definition of hypertension has changed.

○ **How many people in the United States have hypertension?**

Most recent reports indicate that there are 50 million individuals with hypertension.

○ **Is hypertension more common in men or women?**

Women.

○ **What is the definition of hypertension?**

Individuals whose blood pressure exceeds 140 mmHg systolic and/or 90 mmHg diastolic on at least three different examinations.

○ **What should the approach be to treatment of the patient with mild hypertension (diastolic pressure between 90-105 mmHg)?**

Patients with mild diastolic hypertension should be treated, initially with lifestyle modification measures if their diastolic BP is between 90-95 mmHg, and with pharmacologic therapy if diastolic BP exceeds 95 mmHg.

○ **What are some lifestyle modification measures that are effective and should be vigorously stressed in patients with hypertension?**

Weight reduction as close to ideal body weight, sodium restriction, cessation of smoking, moderation of alcohol intake and consistent and regular exercise.

○ **When is pharmacologic therapy indicated in patients with diastolic BP between 90-94 mmHg, even with lifestyle modification?**

Evidence of end-organ involvement, such as LVH, glomerulosclerosis, peripheral vascular disease should prompt pharmacologic therapy, particularly if the patient is black and male and has a strong family history of premature death.

○ **What is the cause of hypertension?**

95% of patients have primary hypertension of undertermined cause. The underlying mechanisms are multifactorial and variable from one patient to another. In general, there is a familial and genetic predisposition that may be associated with metabolic alterations such as sodium sensitivity, carbohydrate intolerance, insulin resistance, hyperuricemia and gout, exogenous obesity, and hyperlipidemia.
5% of patients with hypertension have secondary hypertension.

○ **What are the major secondary causes of hypertension?**

1. Adrenocortical disease, such as Cushing's syndrome, pheochromocytoma and hyperplasia
2. Congenital disorders, such as coarctation of the aorta and adrenal steroidal enzyme defects
3. Drugs, such as corticosteroids, oral contraceptives, NSAIDs, sympathomimetics, narcotics and cocaine use, erythropoietin, and cyclosporine.
4. Neurological disorders, such as increased intracranial pressure and peripheral neuropathy.
5. Renovascular disease, such as renal artery atherosclerosis, renal artery embolization, radiation fibrosis.renal parenchymal disease, both focal and bilateral, as well as polycystic disease.
6. Chronic alcoholism.
7. Post-cardiovascular surgery or post-cardiac transplant surgery.

○   **What is the hemodynamic hallmark of hypertension?**

Increased total peripheral resistance, more or less uniformly distributed throughout the organ circulations.

○   **What two primary cardiovascular adaptations result from the progression of hypertensive disease?**

First, the heart and vessels respond structurally to increased wall stress, thereby increasing left ventricular mass and vascular wall thickness. Second, intravascular volume contracts in most non-volume dependent forms of hypertension in proportion to the increased pressure and vasoconstriction. In addition, plasma renin activity rises in proportion to the contraction of plasma volume.

○   **In advanced hypertension, what effects on the cardiovascular take place?**

When the heart and vessels no longer can adapt structurally and functionally, cardiac failure develops. Secondary hormonal mechanisms come into play, such as the systemic and local cardiac and vascular renin-angiotensin-aldosterone systems, catecholamines, vasopressin, endothelin and atrial natriuretic factor. This results in intravascular volume expansion, impaired renal excretory function and further systemic vasoconstriction.

○   **What is the significance of left ventricular hypertrophy as it relates to cardiovascular morbidity and mortality?**

LVH is an independent risk factor for premature cardiac death, both from ischemic heart disease and arrhythmogenic sudden cardiac death.

○   **What antihypertensive agents can reverse LVH within a few weeks of their use?**

Centrally active adrenergic inhibitors, beta-adrenergic receptor blocking agents, ACE inhibitors and calcium channel antagonists.

○   **If the presence of LVH confers increased risk of premature cardiovascular morbidity and mortality, can the reduction of LVH by pharmacological means reduce the risk associated with it?**

To date, no evidence demonstrating that reducing LVH reduces the cardiovascular risk exists.

○   **What are the types of nonatherosclerotic fibrotic renovascular diseases that can produce hypertension?**

The most frequent is medial fibroplasia ("string of beads" type of lesion). It is most common in women and commonly bilateral. This fibrosing lesion progresses slowly, and the hypertension may not be as severe as in patients with intimal fibroplasia, perimedial fibroplasia or fibromuscular fibroplasia. The latter three fibrosing lesions are more severely stenosing, are associated with more severe elevation in arterial pressure, and are accompanied by the x-ray findings of collateral circulation. Elevation of arterial pressure in these patients is due to the activation of the renin-angiotensin system and the generation of angiotensin

II. Untreated renal artery stenosis can lead to autonephrectomy from total occlusion of the affected renal artery.

○ **What clinical scenarios should strongly raise suspicion of a renovascular component or cause of hypertension?**

1. Sudden development of hypertension or the unexplained increased severity of essential hypertension in any individual (especially the young or elderly).
2. Hypertension in a previously normotensive individual without a family history of hypertension.
3. Appearance of hypertension associated with a renal arterial bruit.
4. Development of drug-resistant hypertension.

○ **What is the treatment of renovascular hypertension?**

Usually medical, but renal artery balloon angioplasty is moderately successful in well-selected patients with renal artery stenosis. Medical therapy must achieve adequate blood pressure reduction while preserving renal function.

○ **What organ is the most irreversibly affected by hypertension?**

The kidneys. While the incidence of stroke, heart failure, dissecting aortic aneurysm, hypertensive encephalopathy and accelerated and malignant hypertension have all been dramatically reduced since the inception of antihypertensive therapy, end-stage renal disease has not diminished. In fact, the number of patients with hypertension who require renal dialysis continues to increase, most notably in black patients.

○ **Ideal antihypertensive therapy should achieve its goals with what features in mind?**

1. The agent reduces vascular smooth muscle tone in order to reduce total peripheral and organ vascular resistance.
2. The agent maintains normal cardiac output and organ blood flows, especially to the heart, kidneys, and brain.
3. The agent does not inordinately stimulate the heart to increase its rate, contractility or metabolism.
4. The agent does not expand intravascular volume in response to the reduced hydrostatic and renal perfusion pressures.

○ **What are the most common symptoms related to early "target organ" involvement from hypertension?**

Decreased exercise tolerance, fatigue, palpitations, rapid or irregular heart rhythm, and nocturia. Chest discomfort, most likely of cardiac origin, may occur as a manifestation of increased myocardial oxygen demand associated with elevated systolic pressure, especially if LVH and/or coexistent coronary artery disease is present.

○ **What are the four stages of hypertensive retinopathy?**

Stage I: increased arterial tortuosity and mild vasoconstriction.
Stage II: arteriovenous nicking, the discontinuity of the arterioles at arteriovenous crossings.
Stage III: appearance of exudates and hemorrhages, representing accelerated hypertension
Stage IV: papilledema, the hallmark of malignant hypertension.

○ **What is the significance of diastolic timing renal bruits?**

They are highly suggestive of renovascular hypertension.

○ **What is the most common cardiac auscultatory finding in patients with hypertension?**

An S4 gallop, due to reduced left ventricular compliance from hypertrophy and collagen deposition.

○   What is Gaisbock's syndrome?

Elevated hemoglobin (polycythemia) related to increasing arterial pressure and total peripheral resistance produced by contracted plasma volume.

○   What percentage of patients with hypertension will eventually develop diabetes mellitus?
Approximately 25-40%.

○   What percentage of patients with diabetes mellitus have, or will develop, hypertension?

Approximately 50-75%.
○   What is the significance of serum uric acid concentration in patients with hypertension?

The higher the serum uric acid in the untreated patient with hypertension, the lower the renal blood flow and the higher the renal vascular resistance. This rise in serum uric acid levels is a marker for the early development of left ventricular hypertrophy and provides evidence that renal vascular involvement in hypertension follows adaptive cardiac changes.

○   What is the basic laboratory evaluation in the uncomplicated hypertensive patient?

If possible, laboratory studies should be obtained with the patient off all medications for at least two weeks. Furthermore, the patient should not be on a sodium-restricted diet for at least two weeks so as not to stimulate the adrenal cortex sufficiently to suggest the possibility of primary aldosteronism. The laboratory evaluation should consist of a CBC, complete urinalysis, determination of serum creatinine and blood urea nitrogen, serum electrolytes, blood glucose, serum uric acid, serum lipid profile, serum calcium and an ECG. A CXR should also be obtained on all patients with hypertension to assess cardiac size and identify pulmonary congestion or aortic enlargement.

○   What is the earliest electrocardiographic sign of cardiac organ involvement from hypertension?

Left atrial enlargement, signifying the first ECG sign of left ventricular hypertrophy. It is often present even in the absence of ECG criteria of LVH.

○   What is the usefulness of 24-hour ambulatory blood pressure monitoring?

1.   Relating clinical condition and target organ involvement to 24-hour pressures.
2.   Clarifying episodic problems such as fluctuations in pressures.
3.   Reconciling office and home pressures with the clinical situation.
4.   Proving adequacy of 24-hour control of pressure with drug therapy.
A lower cost alternative is to have the patient obtain home blood pressure records over a period of time.

○   Which patients are more suitable for diuretic therapy to achieve adequate treatment of hypertension?

Elderly patients, blacks, those patients with volume-dependent forms of hypertension (e.g., expanded intravascular volume, lower plasma renin activity), steroid-dependent forms of hypertension or patients with renal parenchymal disease.

○   Which patients are more amenable to beta-adrenergic receptor blocking monotherapy?

Younger patients (those with greater adrenergic activity), black patients, patients with cardiac arrhythmias or palpitations, patients with angina pectoris or prior myocardial infarction, patients with coexisting diseases that are also amenable to beta-blockers (e.g., migraine headaches, mitral valve prolapse, aortic aneurysm), and patients with hyperdynamic circulation.

O   Which groups of hypertensive patients are more amenable to alpha-adrenergic receptor blocking agents?

Those patients with benign prostatic hypertrophy, those patients intolerant of diuretic therapy, and those incompletely responsive to beta-blockers and/or diuretics, particularly black patients.

O   What is the major side effect of the alpha-1 receptor blockers (e.g., prazosin)? Major drawback?

Postural dizziness secondary to transient postural hypotension. Their major drawback is that they tend to lose effectiveness over time.

O   What is the major drawback to the centrally acting adrenergic-inhibiting drugs, such as clonidine?

Rebound hypertension upon withdrawl or missing doses. This rebound hypertension can be profound.

O   What is the major drawback to the use of direct-acting smooth muscle vasodilators, such as hydralazine?

In response to vasodilation, reflexive cardiovascular stimulation occurs, resulting in increases in heart rate, contractility and metabolism. Thus, angina pectoris, myocardial infarction, further dissection of an aneurysm or overt cardiac failure may be precipitated in the predisposed patient by these agents, either alone or with diuretics.

O   What are the major cardiac advantages of ACE inhibitors in antihypertensive usage?

No reflex cardiac stimulation (no increase in HR, contractility or cardiac output), regression of LVH and left ventricular mass, inhibition of myocardial remodeling after myocardial infarction, and they diminish the amount of accumulated collagen in the ventricle.

O   What are the most common side effects of ACE inhibitors?

Dry cough, rash, loss of taste, hyperkalemia, renal failure in patients with bilateral renal artery disease, and rarely, neutropenia at very high doses. The side effects disappear completely with the cessation of the medication and may not reappear if therapy is resumed with the same agent or another ACE inhibitor.

O   Which patients may be more suitable for initial therapy with ACE inhibitors?

1. Patients with more severe hypertension requiring many antihypertensive agents.
2. Patients who have experienced suboptimal control of pressure with other agents.
3. Patients with essential hypertension with high plasma renin activity or renal artery disease.
4. Patients with cardiac failure or dilated cardiomyopathy.
5. Patients with previous metabolic or other side effects from prior antihypertensive treatment programs.
6. Patients with diabetic nephropathy.

O   Which patients might be expected to respond well to calcium channel antagonists?

1. Patients who also respond well to diuretics.
2. Black patients and elderly patients.
3. Patients with coronary artery disease who cannot take beta-blockers.
4. Patients with bilateral renal artery stenosis or unilateral renal vascular disease who cannot tolerate ACE inhibitors.

○   **A patient with a psychiatric history taking an MAO inhibitor has ingested a 12-pack of beer with a meal of pickled herring and a nice aged cheese. He complains of severe headache. On exam, BP is elevated. A diagnosis of acute hypertension is made secondary to hyperstimulation of the adrenergic receptors. What is the preferred treatment?**

An alpha- and beta-adrenergic antagonist such as labetalol.

○   **What drug can be used for all hypertensive emergencies?**

Sodium nitroprusside (not DOC for eclampsia). Sodium nitroprusside works through production of c-GMP, which relaxes smooth muscle. This results in decreased preload and afterload, decreased oxygen demand, slight increased heart rate with no change in myocardial blood flow, cardiac output, or renal blood flow. Duration of action is 1 to 2 min. Sometimes, beta-blockade is required to treat rebound tachycardia.

○   **What is the most common complication of nitroprusside?**

Hypotension. Thiocyanate toxicity with blurred vision, tinnitus, change in mental status, muscle weakness, and seizures is seen more often in patients with renal failure and after prolonged infusions. Cyanide toxicity is uncommon, it may occur with hepatic dysfunction, after prolonged infusions, and in rates greater than 10 µg/kg per minute.

○   **What is the most common type of secondary hypertension found in the United States?**

Chronic renal disease and renovascular diseases.

○   **What percentage of hypertension is caused by oral contraceptive use?**

Anywhere from 0.2-1.0%.

○   **Among hypertensive patients, does the presence of obesity increase or decrease the risk of coronary mortality?**

Decrease.

○   **Among obese patients, does the presence of hypertension increase or decrease the risk of developing coronary artery disease?**

Increase.

○   **What is an increasingly common contributor to the development of hypertension in obese patients?**

Sleep apnea.

○   **What clinical subsets of patients would create a moderate degree of suspicion for renovascular hypertension and would strongly compel a non-invasive workup for renovascular hypertension?**

1.   Severe hypertension (diastolic blood pressure greater than 120 mm Hg).
2.   Hypertension refractory to standard therapy.
3.   Hypertension with a suggestive abdominal bruit (long, high-pitched and localized to the region of the renal artery.
4.   Abrupt onset of sustained, moderate to severe hypertension at age <20 or age >50.

5. Moderate hypertension (diastolic blood pressure > 105 mm Hg) in a smoker, in a patient with evidence of occlusive vascular disease (cerebrovascular, coronary, peripheral vascular), or in a patient with unexplained but stable elevation of serum creatinine.
6. Normalization of blood pressure by an angiotensin-converting enzyme inhibitor in a patient with moderate or severe hypertension (particularly in a smoker or a patient with recent onset of hypertension.).

O **What clinical subsets of patients would there by a high degree of suspicion for renovascular hypertension and would require either a non-invasive or invasive (arteriography) workup for renovascular hypertension?**

1. Severe hypertension (diastolic blood pressure greater than 120 mm Hg with either progressive renal insufficiency or refractoriness to aggressive treatment particularly in a patient who has been a smoker or has other evidence of occlusive arterial disease).
2. Accelerated or malignant hypertension (grade III or IV retinopathy).
3. Hypertension with recent elevation of serum creatinine, either unexplained or reversibly induced by an ACE inhibitor.
4. Moderate to severe hypertension with incidentally detected asymmetry of renal size by ultrasound or CT scan.

O **What are the indications for surgery in patients with renovascular hypertension?**

Those patients whose hypertension is not well controlled or whose renal function has deteriorated on medical therapy; those patients with only a transient response to renal artery angioplasty; and, those patients whose renal artery lesions are not amenable to angioplasty.

O **What percentage of patients with renovascular hypertension will improve with renal artery angioplasty?**

60-70%, more with fibromuscular disease than with atherosclerosis.

O **What are the clinical conditions that require rapid treatment of hypertension?**

1. Accelerated-malignant hypertension, with or without papilledema
2. Hypertensive encephalopathy
3. Atherothrombotic CVA with severe hypertension
4. Intracerebral hemorrhage or subarachnoid hemorrhage
5. Acute aortic dissection
6. Acute left ventricular failure
7. Acute or impending myocardial infarction
8. Moderate to severe hypertension following coronary artery bypass surgery
9. Acute glomerulonephritis
10. Renal crises from collagen vascular diseases
11. Severe hypertension after renal transplantation
12. Crisis from pheochromocytoma
13. Food or drug interactions with MAO inhibitors
14. Eclampsia
15. Severe hypertension from cocaine or other sympathomimetic drug use
16. Severe hypertension in patients requiring immediate surgery
17. Postoperative hypertension
18. Postoperative bleeding from vascular suture lines
19. Hypertension in a patient with severe body burns
20. Severe epistaxis

O **What are the clinical characteristics of hypertensive crisis?**

1. Blood pressure over 130 mm Hg diastolic

2. Headache, confusion, somnolence, stupor visual loss, focal neurologic deficits, seizures, coma
3. Hemorrhages, exudates, or papilledema on funduscopic exam
4. Prominent apical impulse, cardiac enlargement or congestive heart failure on cardiac exam
5. Oliguria and/or azotemia on renal evaluation
6. Nausea and vomiting

○   **Review the following individual choices of antihypertensive therapy in patients with coexisting conditions.**

Coexisting condition	Diuretic	Beta-blocker	Alpha-blocker	Ca Blocker	ACE inhibitor
Older age (>65)	++	+/-	+	+	+
African-American race	++	+/-	+	+	+/-
Angina	+/-	++	+	++	+
Post MI	+	++	+	+/-*	++
CHF	++	+/-	+	—	++
Cerebrovascular disease	+	+	+/-	++	+
Renal insufficiency	++	+/-	+	++	++
Diabetes Mellitus	+/-	+/-	++	+	++
Hyperlipidemia	—	+/-	++	+	+
Asthma or COPD	+	—	+	++	+
BPH			++		

++ = strongly preferred; + = suitable; +/- = usually not preferred; — = usually contraindicated;
 * = dihydropyridines may be contraindicated; ACEI = angiotensin-converting enzyme inhibitors

ECHOCARDIOGRAPHY AND CARDIAC IMAGING

○ **Doppler flow velocity measure what hemodynamic feature?**

Flow velocity, which is used to calculate pressure gradients across valves and across anatomic structures within the heart and blood vessels. It is not used to assess blood flow.

○ **What echocardiographic view is best to correctly assess the presence of mitral valve prolapse?**

The 2- chamber view is probably the most reliable and has the least false positives. The parasternal long axis view is next best. The apical 4-chamber view is fraught with the most false positives.

○ **What does the maximum instantaneous gradient (MIG) across a valve tell you about the severity of stenotic aortic valves?**

It is not a measure of mean pressure gradient, but it does correlate in a parallel fashion to the mean pressure gradient. MIG's over 50 mmHg are found in severe aortic stenosis.

○ **What is the most accurate view for assessing LV systolic function, both globally and regionally?**

The parasternal short axis view is the best because it looks at a cross-section of all the walls of the LV simultaneously. However, it sometimes is the most difficult to image.

○ **A 74 year-old man prsents with CHF. Physical exam reveals a grade II/VI systolic murmur over the left precordium. Carotid pulse is of low volume with delayed peak. The electrocardiogram shows left bundle branch block. CXR shows moderate cardiomegaly and pulmonary venous congestion. Two-dimensional echocardiography reveals a moderately dilated left ventricular cavity, calcified aortic valve and an LVEF of 25%. The transvalvular peak velocity by continuous wave Doppler is 3.0 m/sec, left ventricular outflow tract velocity is .5 m/sec and the left ventricular outflow diameter is 2.2 cm. The calculated aortic valve area by the continuity equation is .6 cm². What test will provide the best assessment of the severity of aortic stenosis?**

Reassessment of aortic valve with inotropic stimulation.

○ **Which test provides the best information about myocardial viability in the presence of an ischemic cardiomyopathy in a patient with three-vessel disease and a history of myocardial infarction who you are considering for revascularization?**

The best test for myocardial viability is a PET (positron emission tomography) scan. However, they are not readily available to all and they are expensive. The next best test would be a dobutamine stress echocardiography to look for improved contractility in areas of hypokinesis, presumably from hibernating myocardium. A resting thallium scan is also a reasonable test to look for perfusion to areas that are regionally hypokinetic.

○ **What is the best test to diagnose and assess the severity of chronic pulmonary embolism?**

Ultrafast CT of the chest.

❍   What is the formula for calculating the peak pressure gradient across a valve using the flow velocity obtained with continuous wave Doppler flow study?

The pressure gradient across the valve is equal to $4V^2$, where V is the peak flow velocity across the valve sampled. Thus, if the peak velocity across the tricuspid valve is 4 m/second, then the peak gradient across the tricuspid valve is 64 mm Hg.

❍   **How accurate is continuous wave Doppler echocardiography in evaluating the severity of aortic stenosis?**

Very accurate. With technically good images and good acquisition of data using continuous wave Doppler, the aortic valve area, as determined by the continuity equation, can be determined with a high degree of precision and compares very closely with hemodynamic data obtained during cardiac catheterization.

❍   **Why is continuous wave Doppler required to evaluate the severity of valvular heart disease during echocardiography?**

Because pulse wave Doppler cannot sample high velocity blood flow due to aliasing.

❍   **What are the advantages of transesophageal echocardiography over transthoracic echocardiography?**

Transesophageal echocardiography is useful in patients in whom the examination from the usual transthoracic approach is technically difficult or impossible. This approach is particularly useful in assessing prosthetic valves, valvular vegetations, thoracic aortic disease, intracardiac masses and both atrial and ventricular septal defects. Furthermore, the imaging is superior in patients on ventilators, patients with COPD and very obese patients.

❍   **What is the most sensitive and easiest method of detecting right-to-left cardiac shunts?**

Saline contrast echocardiography.

❍   **What is the primary modality used for evaluating left ventricular diastolic function?**

Two-dimensional and M-mode echocardiography.

❍   **What are the changes on echocardiography that suggest diastolic dysfunction?**

Changes seen on the M-mode examination include a decreased E-F slope, a decrease in the early diastolic flow velocity manifested by a decreased E point amplitude, an increase in the late diastolic flow velocity manifested by an increase A point amplitude and a reversal of the E/A ratio from > 1 to < 1. On the Doppler examination, pulse wave early diastolic velocity across the mitral valve becomes diminished and late diastolic velocity across the mitral valve increases. On two-dimensional echo, one can qualitatively see a prolonged relaxation of the left ventricle during diastole.

❍   **What is the earliest sign of coronary artery disease seen on echocardiography?**

Evidence of diastolic dysfunction.

❍   **How can one determine the systolic pulmonary artery pressure using Doppler echocardiography?**

In the presence of tricuspid regurgitation and with no obstruction to blood flow across the right ventricular outflow tract, the peak systolic flow velocity across the tricuspid valve by continuous wave Doppler can be used to accurately assess the systolic pulmonary artery pressure using the formula $P = 4V^2$ where V is the peak flow velocity across the tricuspid valve during systole and P is the pressure gradient. By adding an estimation of the right atrial pressure to the pressure gradient across the tricuspid valve, an accurate estimate of the systolic pulmonary artery pressure is obtained.

○ **What is the pathognomonic finding on M-mode recording of the aortic valve in obstructive hypertrophic cardiomyopathy?**

Mid-systolic closure of the aortic valve.

○ **What is a classic echocardiographic finding on M-mode recording of the mitral valve in aortic regurgitation?**

Diastolic "fluttering" of the anterior leaflet of the mitral valve. It may be accompanied by premature closure of the mitral valve when aortic regurgitation is severe or in acute aortic regurgitation.

○ **Which is more accurate in accurately assessing the severity of valvular regurgitation, echocardiography or cardiac catheterization?**

Cardiac catheterization.

○ **What finding on two-dimensional echocardiography correlates with the presence of an old myocardial infarction?**

Loss of thickening of the myocardium along with increased echodensity of the infarcted myocardial region.

○ **What are the echocardiographic signs of dilated cardiomyopathy?**

Dilated, poorly contracting left ventricular myocardium, poorly moving aorta, reduced opening of the mitral valve and slow closure of the aortic valve.

○ **What are the classic echocardiographic findings in restrictive cardiomyopathy?**

Reduced wall motion and thickening of the left ventricular wall without dilatation. These changes are usually uniform throughout the ventricle.

○ **What are the classic echocardiographic findings in cardiac amyloidosis?**

Left ventricular hypertrophy, an unusually thickened interatrial septum and a sparkling granular or speckled appearance to the myocardium, particularly the septum.

○ **What is the most frequent echocardiographic sign of cardiac tamponade?**

Early diastolic collapse of the right ventricular free wall. Right atrial collapse is more sensitive but less specific.

○ **What imaging technique is the most sensitive and specific for the detection of coronary artery calcification?**

CT scanning.

○ **What is the significance of increase lung uptake of thallium during radionuclide exercise testing?**

It indicates exercise-induced left ventricular dysfunction, presumably from severe myocardial ischemia or poor LV function with exercise-induced heart failure. Transient left ventricular dilatation can also be seen during exercise-induced left ventricular dysfunction.

❍   **What are the characteristic perfusion stress perfusion images in patients with high-risk coronary artery disease?**

1.   Multiple reversible defects in two or more coronary artery territories.
2.   Quantitatively large myocardial perfusion defects.
3.   Increased radiotracer lung uptake after exercise.
4.   Transient dilatation of the left ventricle immediately after exercise.

❍   **Which is more sensitive for establishing the diagnoses of pulmonary embolism, pulmonary angiography or ultrafast CT?**

Ultrafast CT is more sensitive.

EPIDEMIOLOGY AND PREVENTIVE CARDIAC MEDICINE

O   **What are the NCEP adult guidelines regarding the detection of hyperlipidemia?**

All individuals should have a baseline total cholesterol, and, if accuracy can be assured, an HDL cholesterol at age 20, then at least once every five years.

O   **What is the Friedewald formula for calculating LDL cholesterol from measured cholesterol and triglyceride levels obtained from a full fasting lipoprotein analysis?**

LDL cholesterol (mg/dl) = Total cholesterol – HDL cholesterol – (triglyceride/5). The formula is not accurate if triglyceride is greater than 400 mg/dl, if the patient is homozygous for apo-E2 or if the patient has type III hyperlipidemia. LDL cholesterol needs to be measured directly by ultracentrifugation at a specialized laboratory in these instances.

O   **What are the desirable levels of total cholesterol, LDL cholesterol, HDL cholesterol and triglyceride according to NCEP guidelines of primary prevention of CAD?**

Total cholesterol less than 200 mg/dl, LDL cholesterol less than 130 mg/dl, triglyceride less than 200 mg/dl and HDL cholesterol greater than 35 mg/dl.

O   **A 53 year-old African-American male with hypertension and diabetes is referred to you for evaluation of atypical chest pain. He has been well managed on diuretics for hypertension and is taking metformin for his diabetes. His blood sugars have been consistently between 80 and 130 mg/dl. A treadmill test with Technitium imaging revealed no perfusion defects and normal LV systolic function. His fasting lipoprotein analysis revealed the following: total cholesterol 235 mg/dl, triglyceride 175 mg/dl, HDl cholesterol 28 mg/dl, and LDL cholesterol 172 mg/dl. He weighs 225 lbs. and is 69 inches tall. What should his primary prevention strategy consist of?**

Initiate strict diet therapy with a low fat, low cholesterol diet consisting of less than 30% of total caloric intake from fat, no more than 10% of total calories from polyunsaturated fat, no more than 15% of total calories from monounsaturated fat, no more than 8-10% of total calories from saturated fat, cholesterol intake less than 300 mg/day, daily exercise and weight loss to an ideal body weight of between 155 and 170 lbs. A full fasting lipoprotein analysis should be repeated in six months with the goal being a total cholesterol less than 200mg/dl, LDL cholesterol less than 130 mg/dl and an HDL cholesterol greater than 35 mg/dl. One might also consider changing antihypertensive medication from a diuretic to another medication that has either no effect on cholesterol or has a favorable one as long as this patient's blood pressure will continue to be well controlled.

O   **Other than elevated LDL cholesterol, what are the other additional risk factors for coronary artery disease?**

Age (45 years or older in men, 55 years or older in women or premature menopause without estrogen-replacement therapy in women); family history of premature CAD (myocardial infarction or sudden death before age 55 in father or other male first-degree relative, or before the age of 65 in mother or other female first-degree relative); current cigarette smoking; hypertension (greater than or equal to 140/90 mm Hg, or on antihypertensive medication); diabetes mellitus; low HDL cholesterol (<35 mg/dl); obesity.

O   **What is the acceptable blood pressure for the treatment of hypertension in the United States?**

An acceptable level for the reduction of risk factors and end-organ damage is less than 140 mmHg systolic and less than 89 mmHg diastolic. This is especially true for those with heart disease, history of stroke and those with renal disease.

O   **T/F: Triglycerides constitute an independent risk factor for coronary artery disease only in those individuals with obesity.**

False.

O   **T/F: The association between triglycerides and the risk of coronary artery disease has been underestimated since HDL is metabolically inversely related to VLDL.**

True.

O   **In patients with coronary artery disease, what is the optimal LDL cholesterol?**

Below 100 mg/dl.

O   **What is the optimal level of LDL cholesterol in patients without evidence of coronary artery disease, but with two or more risk factors for coronary artery disease?**

Below 130 mg/dl.

O   **What is the optimal level of LDL cholesterol in patients without evidence of coronary artery disease and less than two risk factors for coronary artery disease?**

Below 160 mg/dl.

O   **What is the recommended initial medical therapy in patients with elevated LDL cholesterol and triglycerides over 200 mg/dl?**

Cholestyramine, a combination of cholestyramine and HMG-CoA reductase inhibitor, HMG-CoA reductase inhibitor alone or in combination with niacin or niacin alone are all acceptable choices for initial therapy.

O   **What is the recommended initial medical therapy in patients with elevated LDL cholesterol and triglyceride level between 200-400 mg/dl?**

Niacin, alone or in combination with gemfibrozil or an HMG-CoA reductase inhibitor, is the recommended course.

O   **What is the recommended time frame for checking liver function tests in patients beginning HMG-CoA reductase inhibitors?**

With simvistatin, liver function tests should be checked at 12 weeks, then every 3-6 months thereafter. With lovastatin, liver function tests should be checked at 8 weeks, then every 3-6 months. With atorvastatin, liver function tests should be checked at 6 weeks, then every three months thereafter.

O   **Which is the most potent of the HMG-CoA reductase inhibitors?**

Atorvastatin.

○   **What is the relationship of estrogen hormone replacement and LDL cholesterol, triglycerides, and HDL cholesterol?**

In the first two years, LDL cholesterol and triglyceride levels gradually rise and HDL levels gradually decline. However, after the first two years of therapy, LDL cholesterol and triglyceride levels then decline as much as 15% from baseline levels at the beginning of therapy, and HDL levels rise about 15% above baseline levels.

○   **What is the treatment of patients with isolated high triglyceride levels?**

The primary treatment is lifestyle modification, including weight control, exercise, smoking cessation, alcohol restriction in some patients, and a diet low in saturated fat and cholesterol.

○   **T/F: Omega-3 fatty acids lower triglyceride levels.**

True.

○   **What is the single greatest preventable risk factor for coronary artery disease in the world?**

Cigarette smoking. It multiplies the effect of all other risk factors of coronary artery disease, and alone, is responsible for approximately 20% of all cardiovascular deaths.

○   **Who has a greater adverse effect on cardiovascular risk from cigarette smoking-men or women?**

Women.

○   **Which risk factor for coronary artery disease is probably responsible for the earliest and most severe cases of atherosclerosis?**

Diabetes mellitus.

○   **What is considered the minimum amount of exercise required to achieve a cardioprotective benefit?**

A regular program of 30 minutes of moderate aerobic physical activity three times per week.

○   **Which patients have the highest incidence of fatal myocardial infarction?**

Patients over age 75 years of age.

○   **What other risk factors are associated with increased risk of coronary artery disease?**

Elevated fibrinogen levels, elevated coagulation factor VII, decreased fibrinolytic activity, elevated levels of PAI-1, elevated plasma homocysteine levels, type A personality and stress and low circulating blood concentrations of antioxidants.

CARDIAC CATHETERIZATION AND INTERVENTIONAL CARDIOLOGY

○ **What criteria must be met to confirm the diagnosis of a line infection?**

A series of positive blood cultures and/or a positive line tip culture with greater than 15 colony-forming units with the same organism.

○ **T/F: Single-lumen central venous catheters are less prone to infection.**

True.

○ **What complications are associated with arterial catheterization?**

Thrombosis, infection, pseudoaneurysm and rupture.

○ **What is the treatment for infected vascular catheters?**

Removal of the catheter and, possibly, antibiotic therapy.

○ **What are the most common organisms involved with line infections?**

Staphylococcus epidermidis and *Staphylococcus aureus*.

○ **What are the indications for PTCA?**

Acute evolving MI, critical coronary stenosis, stenotic vein bypass grafts, intraoperative dilatation of distal segmental lesions and distal bypass grafts and patients with 1- or 2-vessel disease.

○ **T/F: Patients with refractory angina and left main CAD should be treated with PTCA?**

False. Significant left main coronary artery disease is a contraindication to PTCA.

○ **What is the restenosis rate within the first six months of PTCA without stenting?**

30-40%.

○ **What is the restenosis rate within the first six months of PTCA with coronary stenting?**

15-20%.

○ **T/F: Stenotic coronary lesions > 2.0 cm long are suitable for PTCA.**

False. If CABG is not feasible or suitable, these lesions are more suitable for atherectomy. The success rate with PTCA for lesions over 2.0 cm long is poor.

○   **T/F: The restenosis rate for proximal LAD lesions is no higher than that for mid- or distal LAD lesions.**

False. As a rule, proximal lesions have a higher restenosis rate than distal lesions, particularly the LAD.

○   **Which revascularization strategy has better results in diabetic patients with 2- or 3-vessel CAD: PTCA or CABG?**

CABG. A much lower reintervention rate over the next three years than patients who underwent PTCA.

○   **What is the long-term success rate for PTCA of vein grafts?**

PTCA of the anastamotic sites in vein grafts is reasonably good with an acceptable restenosis rate of around 30-40%. However, PTCA of the mid-portion of vein grafts has a high restenosis rate and a poor success rate and is generally not advised unless revascularization is absolutely necessary and CABG is not an option.

○   **T/F: The use of non-ionic contrast has a lower rate of nephrotoxicity and post-procedure renal failure than ionic contrast.**

False. The only benefit of non-ionic contrast is a lower rate of allergic and hypersensitivity reactions.

○   **T/F: All coronary stenotic lesions that PTCA is performed on should have coronary stenting?**

False. Only those lesions that are type B or C (less than suitable and more complex for PTCA), and those lesions that have restenosed should have coronary stenting. Type A lesions should not be stented unless there is a compelling reason from a success standpoint.

○   **Following successful resuscitation of patients with sudden cardiac death, what tests must be performed?**

Electrophysiology studies (EPS), cardiac catheterization and coronary angiography.

○   **What is the best view on coronary angiography to assess the proximal LAD and proximal circumflex?**

RAO between 5 and 15 degrees with 25 to 35 degree caudal.

○   **What is the best view on coronary angiography to assess the left main coronary artery?**

LAO at 45-50 degrees with 20 degrees of caudal.

○   **What is the best view to assess the septal perforators?**

LAO at 45 degrees with 15-25 degrees cranial.

○   **What is the rationale for using a catheter with side-holes rather than just an end-hole when performing left ventriculography?**

To minimize the chances of contrast material being injected into the endocardium (endocardial staining).

○   **What is the normal LV end-diastolic volume index on left ventriculography?**

50-90 mm/m^2.

○   **What is the normal LV stroke volume index on left ventriculography?**

35-55 mm/m^2.

○   **What is the normal LV end-systolic volume index on left ventriculography?**

15-35 mm/m^2.

○   **What is the qualitative angiographic classification of mitral regurgitation on left ventriculography?**

1+ (trivial)-contrast opacification enters the left atrium during systole and clears with each beat.
2+ (mild)-contrast opacification enters the left atrium during systole, does not clear with each beat, and is less dense than the opacification of the left ventricle.
3+ (moderate)-contrast opacification enters the left atrium during systole, and is equally dense to that in the left ventricle.
4+ (severe)-contrast opacification occurs in the left atrium in one systolic ejection period, or is more dense than the opacification of the left ventricle, or opacification is seen in a pulmonary vein.

○   **What is the qualitative angiographic classification of aortic regurgitation on central aortography?**

1+ (trivial)-contrast opacification enters the left ventricle during diastole and clears with each beat.
2+ (mild)-contrast opacification enters the left ventricle during diastole, does not clear with each beat, and is less dense than the opacification of the aortic root.
3+ (moderate)-contrast opacification enters the left ventricle during diastole, and is equally dense to that in the central aorta.
4+ (severe)-contrast opacification of the left ventricle is greater than the opacification of the central aorta, or the left ventricle is opacified in one diastolic filling period.

○   **What are the radiographic signs diagnostic of pulmonary embolism?**

A large intraluminal filling defect in one of the pulmonary arteries or an abrupt pulmonary arterial cut-off. Other radiographic signs, such as localized oligemia and asymmetry of pulmonary blood flow, are suggestive but not strictly diagnostic of embolism.

○   **What is the most common adverse event occurring during selective coronary angiography?**

Transient bradycardia and/or hypotension, most commonly with angiography of the right coronary artery.

○   **What is the overall incidence of death during or within 24 hours of a cardiac catheterization?**

0.1 to 0.2%. The majority of these patients have extensive cardiac disease and these deaths are caused by perforation of the heart or great vessels, cardiac arrhythmias, or acute myocardial infarction.

○   **What is the incidence of acute myocardial infarction during or immediately following cardiac catheterization?**

0.3%.

○   **What is the risk of periprocedural death in patients with significant left main coronary artery stenosis who undergo a cardiac catheterization?**

0.86%.

○   **What is the risk of cerebrovascular accidents in patients undergoing cardiac catheterization?**

0.1 to 0.15%. Most of these are embolic in nature.

○   **What are some of the minor complications associated with cardiac catheterization?**

Thrombosis of the artery catheterized (either femoral or brachial, depending on the approach); hemorrhage or hematoma of the site of arterial puncture; local infection; nausea and vomiting from injection of contrast; ventricular irritability, secondary to endocardial injection of contrast; allergic reactions to contrast injection, including anaphylaxis in rare occurrences; and transient renal insufficiency, which may be severe, particularly in patients with pre-existing renal disease and diabetes mellitus.

○   **What is the overall mortality associated with PTCA?**

Around 1%.

○   **What is the success rate of achieving antegrade flow with PTCA in an infarct-related coronary artery when the infarction is less than 12 weeks old?**

75-90%.

○   **What is the success rate of achieving antegrade flow with PTCA in an infarct-related coronary artery when the infarction is more than 12 weeks old, but less than 6 months old?**

10-25%.

○   **What are the Class I indications for coronary angiography in asymptomatic patients with known or suspected coronary artery disease?**

1) Individuals with evidence for high risk on non-invasive testing; 2) individuals in high-risk occupations, such as airline pilots and bus drivers, who need medical clearance for job continuation; and 3) in patients who are cardiac arrest survivors.

○   **What are the Class II indications for coronary angiography in asymptomatic patients with known or suspected coronary artery disease?**

1. Positive noninvasive test in a non-high-risk patient.
2. Multiple risk factors for coronary artery disease.
3. Prior MI with positive noninvasive testing.
4. Following cardiac transplantation.
5. In patients who have undergone CABG or PTCA with documented ischemia on noninvasive testing or electrocardiography.
6. In patients who are undergoing noncardiac surgery with a positive noninvasive test for ischemia.

○   **What are the Class I indications for coronary angiography in patients with symptomatic coronary artery disease?**

1. Inadequate response to maximal medical therapy.
2. Unstable angina.
3. Prinzmetal's or variant angina.
4. Canadian Class I or II angina associated with the following:

- Positive exercise test.
- History of MI or hypertension with ECG changes.
- Intolerable side effects of medical therapy.
- Occupational or lifestyle "need to know".
- Episodic pulmonary edema.

5.   Before major vascular surgery if angina is present or patient has positive noninvasive testing for ischemia.
6.   Symptomatic patients who have survived cardiac arrest.

○   **What are the Class I indications for coronary angiography in patients with atypical chest pain of uncertain origin?**

1.   When noninvasive stress testing reveals high risk for coronary artery disease.
2.   Suspected coronary artery aneurysm.
3.   Associated symptoms or signs of abnormal LV function or failure in patients with atypical chest pain.

○   **What are the Class II indications for coronary angiography in symptomatic patients with known or suspected coronary artery disease?**

1.   Patients with angina under the age of 40 with either a positive noninvasive test or prior MI.
2.   Patients requiring major nonvascular surgery.
3.   Class 3 or 4 angina that improves on medical therapy.
4.   Patients who cannot be risk-stratified by other techniques.

○   **What are the Class II indications for coronary angiography in patients with atypical chest pain of uncertain origin?**

In patients in whom coronary artery disease cannot be excluded by noninvasive studies, and in patients who have severe symptoms despite negative noninvasive studies.

○   **What are the Class I indications for coronary angiography in patients with completed myocardial infarction prior to discharge from the hospital (after 6 hr and before discharge evaluation)?**

1.   Recurrent episodes of ischemic chest pain.
2.   Suspected ruptured septum or acute mitral regurgitation with CHF.
3.   Suspected left ventricular pseudoaneurysm.

○   **What are the Class II indications for coronary angiography in patients with completed myocardial infarction prior to discharge from the hospital?**

1.   Thrombolytic therapy during evolving MI period.
2.   CHF and/or hypotension during intensive medical therapy.
3.   Recurrent VT and/or VF.
4.   Cardiogenic shock.
5.   MI due to coronary embolism.

○   **What are the Class I indications for coronary angiography in patients with valvular heart disease?**

1.   Before valve surgery in an adult with chest discomfort and/or ECG changes.
2.   Before valve surgery in a male patient age 35 or older.
3.   Before valve surgery in a postmenopausal female patient.

○   **What are the Class II indications for coronary angiography in patients with valvular heart disease?**

1. During left heart catheterization in men age 35 or older, or in women older than 40 when aortic or mitral valve surgery is being contemplated.
2. Patients with valvular heart disease with multiple risk factors for coronary artery disease.
3. Patients who need reoperation for valve surgery when previous coronary angiography is more than 1 year ago.
4. In patients with infective endocarditis when coronary embolization occurs or is suspected.

○   **What are the Class I indications for coronary angiography in patients in the post-discharge period following an acute myocardial infarction (discharge to 8 weeks post-MI)?**

1. Angina at rest or with minimal activity.
2. CHF, recurrent ischemia, or ventricular tachycardia.
3. Positive noninvasive study
4. Non-Q wave infarction.

○   **What are the Class II indications for coronary angiography in patients in the post-discharge period following an acute myocardial infarction (discharge to 8 weeks post-MI)?**

1. Mild angina.
2. Asymptomatic patients under the age of 50.
3. Patients with a need to return to unusually active or vigorous activity.
4. Patients with a previous history of MI or angina for greater than 6 months prior to the current MI.
5. Thrombolytic therapy given during evolving phase.

○   **What are some other Class I indications for coronary angiography?**

1. Disease of the aorta in which the presence or extent of coronary disease will affect the management.
2. Patients with LV failure without obvious cause.
3. Patients with angina associated with hypertrophic cardiomyopathy over age 35.

○   **What are some other Class II indications for coronary angiography?**

1. Patients with dilated cardiomyopathy without obvious cause.
2. Patients with recent blunt chest trauma.
3. Male patients age 35 or older or postmenopausal women about to undergo other cardiac surgery.
4. Prospective transplant donors.
5. Patients with Kawasaki's disease (coronary aneurysms).

○   **What is the mortality rate for coronary angiography in patients with three-vessel CAD?**

0.16%.

○   **What are the indications for the use of non-ionic contrast in coronary angiography?**

Unstable ischemic syndromes, decompensated congestive heart failure, diabetes mellitus, pre-existing renal insufficiency, hypotension, severe bradycardia, history of contrast allergy, severe valvular heart disease, and internal mammary artery injection.

○   **How does one perform left ventriculography in a patient with a mechanical prosthetic mitral and aortic valve?**

Using direct transthoracic left ventricular puncture. This procedure is usually performed with the aide of echocardiography. Retrograde catheterization of the left ventricle across a tilting disc prosthetic aortic valve or transeptal antegrade catheterization of the left ventricle across a tilting disc prosthetic mitral valve are contraindicated due to the risk of catheter entrapment, occlusion of the prosthetic valve, or possible dislodgment of the valve disc with embolization. With the advent of transesophageal echocardiography, this procedure is infrequently performed.

○ **What are the complications and complication rates of endomyocardial biopsy?**

Cardiac perforation with cardiac tamponade is reported to occur less than 0.05%. Cardiac arrhythmias are the most common complication, occurring about 1-2% of cases, but only rarely are they serious. Electrical conduction disturbances, such as bundle branch blocks or complete AV block are quite rare, occurring a reported 0.1-0.3% of cases. Embolization of air, tissue or thrombus is also rare, occurring from 0.1-0.2% of cases. Damage to heart valves and pneumothorax also occur about 0.1-0.2% of the time.

○ **What are the indications for percutaneous intraaortic balloon pump insertion?**

1. Patients with unstable angina, refractory to maximal medical therapy.
2. Patients with cardiogenic shock, secondary to ischemic cardiac events.
3. Patients with mechanical complications of acute myocardial infarction (including severe mitral regurgitation, ventricular septal defect).
4. Patients with severe left main coronary artery stenosis who will be undergoing cardiac surgery.
5. Patients with coronary artery disease undergoing high-risk PTCA and after primary PTCA in the setting of acute myocardial infarction.

○ **What are the complications of percutaneous intraaortic balloon pump insertion?**

Limb ischemia is the most common complication, occurring a reported 12-40%, with most cases resolving upon balloon removal without the need for surgery. Other complications include balloon rupture, balloon entrapment, hematomas and sepsis.

○ **Which factors increase the risk of vascular complications from percutaneous balloon pump insertion?**

Patients with diabetes, patients with pre-existing peripheral vascular disease, female patients, and those patients with a post-insertion ankle-brachial index of less than 0.8.

○ **What percentage of patients undergoing PTCA experience decreased angina following the procedure? Elimination of angina?**

88% and 76%, respectively.

○ **What is the mortality rate for PTCA?**

About 1%. It is 2-3% in the setting of acute myocardial infarction.

○ **What is the incidence of abrupt vessel closure in PTCA?**

Between 4 and 8%.

○ **What is the incidence of myocardial infarction resulting from PTCA-related abrupt vessel closure?**

2-4%.

○ **What is the incidence of emergency CABG needed as a result of PTCA complications?**

2-3%.

○ **What is the major mechanism of abrupt coronary artery closure from PTCA?**

Extensive disruption of the medial layer, leading to obstructive dissection and intramural hematoma, platelet deposition and activation with formation of thrombin, ultimately leading to intracoronary occlusive thrombosis.

O   **What are the pharmacological measures recommended to reduce the incidence of abrupt coronary artery closure?**

Administration of aspirin and administration of a dose of heparin sufficient to increase the activated coagulation time (ACT) to at least 300-350 seconds prior to the first inflation. In patients with suboptimal angiographic results following PTCA, intravenous heparin has been shown to reduce the incidence of post-procedure vessel closure. Recent trials have also shown that administration of c7E3Fab monoclonal antibody fragment, a IIb/IIIa platelet inhibitor also reduces periprocedure vessel closure.

O   **What is the management of abrupt vessel closure in PTCA?**

Typical management consists of repeat prolonged balloon dilatation to induce adhesion of obstructive dissection flaps to the arterial wall, followed by placement of an intracoronary stent.

O   **What are the major factors that have been identified as associated with elevated risk of mortality and morbidity in patients undergoing PTCA?**

Unstable angina, acute myocardial infarction, diabetes mellitus, advanced age, type C lesions, suboptimal angiographic result, and possibly female gender (conflicting studies).

O   **What is the 1-, 5-, and 10-year survival of patients revascularized by PTCA?**

97%, 88-97%, and 78-90% respectively.

O   **What percentage of patients undergoing PTCA will require either repeat PTCA or revascularization with CABG within the first year after the initial PTCA?**

About 15-40%.

O   **What clinical factors increase the likelihood of restenosis following PTCA?**

Unstable angina, variant angina, diabetes mellitus, male gender, cigarette smoking, hyperlipidemia, and end-stage renal disease.

O   **What anatomical factors increase the likelihood of restenosis following PTCA?**

Severe preangioplasty stenosis, proximal stenosis, left anterior descending artery stenosis, long stenosis (>2.0 cm in length), saphenous vein graft stenosis, chronic total occlusion, lesion calcification, bend stenosis, bifurcation stenosis, ostial stenosis, and presence of collaterals.

O   **Which procedural factors increase the likelihood of restenosis following PTCA?**

Postangioplasty residual stenosis > 30%, use of undersized angioplasty balloon, and small residual minimal luminal diameter.

O   **What are the absolute contraindications to PTCA?**

Absence of a hemodynamically significant coronary stenosis, > 50% stenosis of the left main coronary artery which is unprotected by at least one patent bypass graft, and absence of on-site cardiac surgical backup.

○ **What is the optimal time to perform PTCA following successful thrombolytic reperfusion in patients with acute myocardial infarction?**

Between 10-14 days following successful thrombolytic administration in acute myocardial infarction. PTCA done sooner, unless emergent, is associated with a higher mortality rate, higher reocclusion rate, higher recurrent ischemia rate and higher need for emergency CABG, and does not seem to improve ventricular function or long-term outcome.

○ **What is "rescue PTCA" and where is it indicated?**

"Rescue PTCA" is angioplasty performed in the setting of unsuccessful reperfusion with thrombolytic therapy in the setting of acute myocardial infarction. It is most beneficial in large myocardial infarctions, where the post-infarction incidence of death or severe CHF is reduced with "rescue PTCA" from 15-20% down to 5-10%.

○ **T/F: Directional coronary atherectomy is superior to balloon angioplasty in terms of patency rates and restenosis rates.**

False. Directional coronary atherectomy has been shown to have similar vessel patency rates to balloon angioplasty and has a similar restenosis rate (though the trends show a slightly reduced rate with atherectomy).
The complication rates with atherectomy, however, are considerably higher, particularly that of abrupt closure and death.

○ **T/F: Laser angioplasty is superior to balloon angioplasty in terms of patency rate, restenosis rate and complication rates.**

False. Laser angioplasty has similar vessel patency rates and restenosis rates, compared to balloon angioplasty. However, the incidence of complications with laser angioplasty is higher than that of balloon angioplasty, particularly that of coronary dissection and perforation.

CARDIAC SURGERY

O   **What is the major risk factor for prosthetic vascular graft infection?**

Location. The incidence of infection is 1 to 1.5% for aortoiliac grafts as opposed to 2 to 7% for femoral-popliteal arterial grafts.

O   **What are the most common causes of postoperative seizures following aortic valve replacement?**

Air, calcium and atherosclerotic emboli.

O   **What patients have improved longevity with coronary artery bypass grafts (CABG)?**

Those patients with left main coronary artery disease, regardless of LV function and those with 3-vessel disease and depressed LV function (LVEF < 40%). There is also some evidence that patients with 2 vessel disease, where one of the vessels involved is the proximal LAD, has a better outcome with coronary bypass than with PTCA or medical therapy.

O   **What is the main contraindication to CABG?**

Refractory CHF with severe pulmonary hypertension.

O   **What is the mortality rate of patients undergoing CABG?**

Approximately 2%.

O   **What percentage of patients have fewer episodes of angina following CABG?**

90%. Complete resolution is seen in about 75-80% of patients.

O   **What is the risk of infection of a transvenous pacemaker in the first 3 years after insertion?**

1 to 3%.

O   **What risk factors are associated with pacemaker infections?**

Diabetes, malignancy, skin disorders, malnutrition, anticoagulants, steroids and immunosuppressive medications.

O   **What complications are associated with pacemaker insertion?**

Post-insertion hematoma, seroma and infection.

O   **What complications are associated with infected endovascular leads?**

Valvular endocarditis, infected mural thrombi, localized abscesses and electrode perforation.

O   **What organism is most commonly associated with late infections following pacemaker insertion?**

Staphylococcus epidermidis.

O   **In performing repair of an ASD, there is poor decompression of the right heart despite achieving good bypass with bicaval cannulation. What is the most likely diagnosis?**

A persistent left superior vena.

O   **What organism is most commonly associated with infection within the first month of pacemaker insertion?**

Staphylococcus aureus.

O   **What is the preferred approach for repair of most VSD's?**

Transatrial.

O   **What is the most common cause of arrythmias and hypotension during thoracic operations?**

Pericardial manipulation.

O   **Following dacron patch repair of a paramembranous VSD, a patient develops complete heart block. What is the most appropriate next step?**

Epicardial pacing.

O   **What is the most likely location of the conduction system in the above patient?**

Along the posteroinferior border of paramembranous VSD.

O   **What are the indications for ventricular aneurysm resection?**

CHF, recurrent malignant ventricular arrhythmias, angina pectoris and peripheral embolization.

O   **T/F: Preservation of the left anterior descending (LAD) artery is mandatory when resecting a ventricular aneurysm?**

False.

O   **What are the physiologic effects of prolonged extracorporeal circulation?**

Progressive sludging of blood elements in the capillary circulation, RBC hemolysis, coagulation defects, denaturation of plasma proteins and fat emboli.

O   **What postoperative complications are associated with prolonged extracorporeal circulation.**

Bleeding, renal and respiratory insufficiency, focal and general CNS symptoms and pancreatitis.

O   **Postpericardiotomy syndrome occurs in what percentage of patients who have undergone pericardiotomy?**

10 to 30%.

O   **What are the clinical manifestations of the postpericardiotomy syndrome?**

Fever, pericarditis, pleuritis and a pericardial friction rub.

○   **What is the clinical presentation of a prosthetic vascular graft infection?**

Erythema, skin breakdown and purulent drainage.

○   **What is the treatment for prosthetic vascular graft infections?**

Removal of the graft and debridement of the surrounding tissue. Extra-anatomic bypass or amputation may be required.

○   **A 51 year-old male underwent CABG 5 hours ago and suddenly becomes hypotensive with a cardiac index (CI) of 1.5 l/min, central venous pressure (CVP) of 20 mm Hg, left atrial pressure of 24 mm Hg and has significantly increased drainage from his mediastinal thoracostomy tube. What is the treatment of choice?**

Immediate mediastinal re-exploration.

CARDIAC MANAGEMENT OF THE SURGICAL PATIENT

O A 76 year-old gentleman is seen by vascular surgery. The vascular surgeons plan to repair an asymptomatic abdominal aortic aneurysm. The patient's only medical problems are hypertension (treated with a thiazide diuretic), diabetes mellitus (treated with insulin), and degenerative arthritis which limits his ambulation to two blocks. What is the most important test for reducing this patient's perioperative risk?

A thorough history and physical examination. The history should focus on the patient's functional capacity (exercise tolerance), control of his hypertension and diabetes, prior history of bleeding disorders and presence of angina, heart failure or ventricular arrhythmias. Only after a thorough history and physical exam should further laboratory or diagnostic tests be considered.

O In the above patient, what particular findings would you focus on?

Evidence of congestive heart failure, as evidenced by an S3 gallop, jugular venous distension, and bibasilar lung crackles, would carry the greatest risk for a perioperative complication.

O What is the most important test in the assessment of this patient's perioperative risk?

A non-invasive assessment test to assess the presence and severity of coronary artery disease. The most appropriate test in this patient toward this end would be a dipyridamole thallium or technetium myocardial perfusion stress test. Echocardiogram or radionuclide assessment of cardiac function does not appear to confer any additional useful information in the assessment of perioperative risk.

O What is the value of a normal pre-operative ECG in this patient?

Pre-operative ECG's are poor predictors of the presence of coronary artery disease, but they are useful in predicting the perioperative prognosis in the non-vascular surgical patient. In the patient undergoing vascular surgery, however, the ECG is a poor predictor of outcome, even when normal. A normal pre-operative ECG in a patient undergoing non-vascular surgery generally confers a favorable perioperative outcome.

O What would be an alternative to pharmacological stress testing in the assessment of this patient?

If this patient had a contraindication to pharmacological stress testing, coronary angiography at the time of aortography would be appropriate.

O A 65 year-old man is about to undergo an elective repair of a torn medial collateral ligament of the right thumb. After completing a normal history and physical exam, what additional laboratory evaluations would you order?

This patient has a very low cardiopulmonary risk for surgery. Other than a pre-operative ECG, no further tests are necessary.

O The above patient has a pre-operative ECG that reveals LBBB. What are your recommendations?

The presence of LBBB in an asymptomatic patient with a normal history and physical exam does not increase his perioperative risk. Furthermore, no thought should be given to the placement of a temporary transvenous pacemaker as his risk of developing complete AV block in the perioperative period is very low.

O   **What is the perioperative mortality in the first 48 hours for a healthy patient undergoing general anesthesia?**

The estimated mortality in the first 48 hours after surgery in a healthy patient is about 0.1-0.3%. Of all the deaths, 10% occur during anesthesia induction, 35% occur intraoperatively and 55% occur in the remaining 48 hours.

O   **What is the most common cause of perioperative complications in patients undergoing vascular surgery?**

Acute myocardial infarction.

O   **In a patient with a prior myocardial infarction, when is it safe to perform an elective surgical procedure?**

Waiting at least 6 months after an acute myocardial infarction is advised before performing any elective surgical procedure. This applies to both Q wave and non-Q wave myocardial infarctions. With careful patient selection and aggressive perioperative hemodynamic monitoring, some patients may undergo surgery after 3 months following an acute myocardial infarction. For patients needing coronary artery bypass surgery following an acute myocardial infarction, the optimal waiting time is at least 14 days.

O   **When do most perioperative myocardial infarctions occur?**

Most occur postoperatively. Non-Q wave infarctions tend to occur within the first 48 hours following surgery, while Q wave infarctions tend to occur between the third and seventh postoperative day.

O   **What is the most common symptom of perioperative myocardial infarction in an elderly patient?**

In the elderly, more than 50% of perioperative infarctions are NOT accompanied by typical angina. Any postoperative complaint of dyspnea, unexplained tachycardia, hypotension, new onset congestive heart failure, new onset dysrrhythmia, or change in mental status should raise the clinical suspicion of a perioperative myocardial infarction.

O   **What are the most common causes of death within the first 48 hours of surgery?**

In decreasing order of frequency, myocardial infarction, peritonitis, congestive heart failure, sepsis, and pulmonary embolism.

O   **A 72 year-old male is scheduled for elective abdominal aortic aneurysm repair. On the evening prior to this patient's surgery, his ECG shows occasional premature ventricular contractions. The anesthesiologist is concerned that the patient may go into ventricular tachycardia and asks for a cardiology consult. What do you recommend?**

Asymptomatic PVC's do NOT require treatment. The general rule of thumb for pre-operative rhythm disturbances is to treat only those dysrrhythmias that would ordinarily be treated even if the patient were not going to surgery.

O   **In the above patient, the ECG also shows RBBB and left anterior fascicular block. What are your recommendations?**

Asymptomatic bifascicular block does not require treatment. The risk of developing acute complete heart block during surgery is less than 1%. Temporary pacemakers are indicated only in those situations that would warrant permanent pacing outside of the perioperative setting.

○ **Which is safer in high-risk cardiac patients – general anesthesia or spinal anesthesia?**

Neither. Spinal or epidural anesthesia has not been shown to be safer alternatives than general anesthesia in patients with high-risk cardiac conditions.

○ **Which valvular heart disease is associated with the highest perioperative complication rate?**

Aortic stenosis.

○ **What two risk factors, when present, carry the highest cardiac risk in patients undergoing non-cardiac surgery?**

Congestive heart failure and previous myocardial infarction in the last 6 months prior to surgery.

○ **A 71 year-old gentleman is scheduled for an elective carotid endarterectomy. He has a long history of hypertension and his pre-operative BP is 185/115 mmHg. How would you manage his hypertension pre-operatively?**

The surgery should be postponed and his blood pressure should be adequately reduced over the next several weeks with judicious antihypertensive medication adjustments. Rapidly lowering this patient' s blood pressure just prior to surgery can actually increase this patient's perioperative risk.

○ **What is the best antihypertensive agent to use to treat elevated blood pressure in a patient scheduled for aortic aneurysm repair?**

Beta-blockers.

○ **What is the major perioperative risk in a patient with hypertension?**

The most important perioperative risk in a hypertensive patient is the potential for wide variations in blood pressure. A 50% drop in blood pressure at anytime perioperatively or a 33% drop in blood pressure sustained for 10 minutes or longer is associated with a 15-20% incidence of cardiac complications, such as myocardial infarction and congestive heart failure.

○ **What is the best management strategy for a type I diabetic patient presenting with diabetic ketoacidosis and an acute abdomen?**

Diabetic ketoacidosis can mimic the signs of an acute abdomen and it is best to delay surgery for at least 4-6 hours in order to correct fluid and electrolyte disorders as much as possible to reduce perioperative morbidity and mortality.

○ **What associated physical exam findings may place the diabetic patient at particularly high risk for perioperative complications?**

Autonomic neuropathy. These patients have wide blood pressure swings during and after surgery and need to be closely monitored.

○ **A 55 year-old black male with chronic renal failure is in need of coronary artery bypass surgery. What pre-operative tests are important to assess this patient's risk of surgery?**

Aside from the usual pre-operative history and physical examination, CBC, electrolytes and ECG, a bleeding time is very useful. Patients with chronic renal failure frequently have markedly prolonged bleeding times and are prone to intra-operative and post-operative hemorrhage.

O   **A 51 year-old black female with severe coronary artery disease is referred for coronary artery bypass surgery. She is a Jehovah's witness, and according to her religious beliefs, will not allow any blood transfusions or even autotransfusions during or after surgery. Can she be safely operated on and what preoperative measures can be undertaken to lower her risk?**

Patients who refuse blood transfusion, for any reason, can be safely revascularized with bypass surgery, provided their preoperative hemoglobin is slightly higher than that for other selected patients. Optimal hemoglobin levels for such a patient should be between 15-17 for men and between 13-15 for women. This can be accomplished with the administration of erythropoietin three times per week for 3-4 weeks prior to surgery. Volume support can be accomplished perioperatively with intravenous crystalloid.

O   **What is the most common cause of death in patients with chronic renal failure undergoing elective surgery?**

Sepsis and acute myocardial infarction.

O   **A patient with a history of peripartum cardiomyopathy with two children is referred to you for cardiac evaluation after her second delivery. She suffered congestive heart failure during the terminal stages of her pregnancy, but had an uneventful delivery and resolution of her symptoms. She has no exertional limitations at present and denies orthopnea or PND. What should your advice be towards any further pregnancies?**

She should be advised to seek elective sterilization as her risk of congestive heart failure and permanent dilated cardiomyopathy is high with any subsequent pregnancies.

O   **Which patients are at risk for peripartum cardiomyopathy?**

Peripartum cardiomyopathy occurs in 1 in 10,000 in the United States. Women with twin pregnancies, over 30, African-American women and multiparous women are at increased risk.

O   **What percentage of women with peripartum cardiomyopathy recover?**

50-60% of women demonstrate complete or near-complete recovery within six months post partum. The remainder of patients demonstrate either continuous clinical deterioration, leading to cardiac transplantation or early death, or persistent left ventricular dysfunction and chronic heart failure.

O   **What is the management strategy in patients with peripartum cardiomyopathy?**

Similar to those with dilated cardiomyopathy and chronic congestive heart failure, except that ACE inhibitors cannot be safely used. Hydralazine, as an afterload-reducing agent, can be safely used in pregnancy. Because of the increased incidence of thromboembolic events in these patients, anticoagulation with heparin is strongly recommended during pregnancy.

O   **What is the recommended antihypertensive agent in pregnancy?**

Methyldopa has the best and longest track record and is recommended as first line agent. Beta-blockers and hydralazine are useful, both in combination with methyldopa and as alternatives.

O   **A 63 year-old patient of yours with chronic atrial fibrillation, treated with coumadin, is scheduled for an elective inguinal hernia repair. How long should he stop coumadin prior to surgery and when can he resume taking coumadin?**

Coumadin should be stopped 4-5 days prior to surgery and can be started back at the same dose 24 hours after surgery.

O   **Another patient of yours with chronic atrial fibrillation and a mitral valve mechanical prosthesis is also scheduled for inguinal hernia surgery the same day. How long should he stop coumadin prior to surgery and what should his preoperative strategy be?**

Patients with mechanical prosthetic valves in the mitral position are at increased risk for valve thrombosis and thromboembolic events perioperatively. This patient should stop his coumadin and be given low-molecular weight heparin as an outpatient for 5 days prior to surgery, stopping it 6 hours prior to surgery. 12-24 hours after surgery, he should be restarted on full dose intravenous regular or low-molecular weight heparin (enoxaprin) to therapeutic APPT levels of 2-3 times normal and resume coumadin 1-2 days after surgery until his INR is back to between 2.0 and 3.0. Then, his heparin can be stopped.

O   **In a patient with a past history of endocarditis, what prophylasix would you recommend prior to a Cesarean section?**

No prophylaxis is required for this patient.

O   **In a patient with a past history of endocarditis, what prophylaxis would you recommend prior to a vaginal hysterectomy?**

Either amoxicillin 3.0 grams orally one hour before the procedure and then 1.5 grams 6 hours after the initial dose. Alternatively, one can give intravenous ampicillin 2.0 grams plus gentamicin 1.5 mg/kg (not to exceed 80mg), 30 minutes before the operation, which may be repeated 8 hours after the initial dose. Penicillin-allergic patients can be given Vancomycin 1 gram intravenously over 1 hour prior to the operation instead of oral ampicillin or intravenous amoxicillin.

O   **You receive a call from a dentist who is ready to perform several tooth extractions on your 65 year-old patient that had coronary artery bypass surgery 6 months ago. What antibiotic prophylaxis would you recommend?**

No prophylaxis is required for patients with prior coronary artery bypass surgery.

O   **An 81 year-old gentleman presents to your emergency room with near-syncope and is found to be in complete AV block. You schedule him for a permanent pacemaker implantation for tomorrow. What antibiotic prophylaxis would you recommend for this patient?**

Cefazolin (Ancef) 1-2 grams intravenously, just prior to the operation.

O   **What antibiotic regimen would you recommend for a patient with mitral regurgitation and hypertrophic cardiomyopathy about to have an elective colectomy for ulcerative colitis?**

Oral neomycin 1 gram and erythromycin 1 gram every 8 hours for 3 doses the day before surgery.

O   **A 25 year-old Hispanic female with severe rheumatic mitral stenosis is referred to you because of increased shortness of breath and fatigue. She is 28 weeks pregnant. On physical exam, she is in mild congestive heart failure. Her heart rhythm sounds regular on auscultation. What are your recommendations to her obstetrician?**

She should be started on lasix to correct her pulmonary edema. She should be advised to rest and not perform any strenuous activity throughout the remainder of her pregnancy. Since labor presents a significant strain on the cardiovascular system, thought to caesarean section must be seriously considered, although most patients can safely deliver vaginally. The onset of atrial fibrillation or flutter must be aggressively treated with heart rate reduction with the use of beta-blockers and/or digoxin, both of which can be safely used in pregnancy. Anticoagulation with subcutaneous heparin, while not absolutely safe, is recommended for patients in atrial fibrillation as coumadin cannot be taken safely. Heparin must be stopped at the onset of labor.

○   **What are some of the hemodynamic changes seen during normal pregnancy?**

Progressive increases in blood volume, heart rate and cardiac output throughout pregnancy, increases in stroke volume and pulse pressure in early to mid pregnancy, a fall in diastolic blood pressure and systemic vascular resistance in early to mid-pregnancy and little or no change in systolic blood pressure.

○   **What normal auscultatory findings occur in pregnancy?**

Most pregnant women develop a mid-systolic flow murmur best heard at the left sternal border and pulmonic area by the second trimester, which may get louder as the pregnancy continues to term. A venous hum, heard over the right supraclavicular area is also common. An increased S1 sound with exaggerated splitting and a persistent split S2 sound are also common. Diastolic murmurs are rare.

○   **Does pregnancy increase the incidence of arrhythmias?**

Yes. Atrial fibrillation and atrial flutter are more common in pregnancy than in non-pregnant women of childbearing age. Complete heart block, usually congenital, is also occasionally seen.

○   **Can permanent pacemakers be implanted in pregnancy?**

Yes, with electrocardiographic or echocardiographic guidance in order to avoid ionizing radiation exposure to the fetus.

○   **What conditions predispose to peripartum acute myocardial infarction?**

Pheochromocytoma, collagen vascular disease, Kawasaki's disease and sickle cell anemia.

○   **What is the coronary angiogram of a patient with peripartum acute myocardial infarction likely to show?**

Usually normal coronary arteries or coronary artery dissection.

○   **What is the management strategy in patients with peripartum acute myocardial infarction?**

Anti-ischemic medial management with beta-blockers and low-dose aspirin can be safely employed. In patients with hemodynamic instability or recurrent ischemia, serious consideration to termination of the pregnancy must be given. Non-invasive myocardial perfusion testing and coronary angiography should only be used when absolutely necessary due to the unknown effects of ionizing radiation on the fetus.

○   **Which cardiac medications are safe in pregnancy?**

Digoxin, quinidine, lidocaine, adenosine, beta-blockers and hydralazine. Other agents such as nitrates, diuretics, and calcium channel antagonists are safe but must be used with caution. Coumadin, amiodarone, nitroprusside and ACE inhibitors should be avoided due to adverse fetal events.

CARDIAC GRAPHICS

○ **What is the cardiac arrhythmia?**

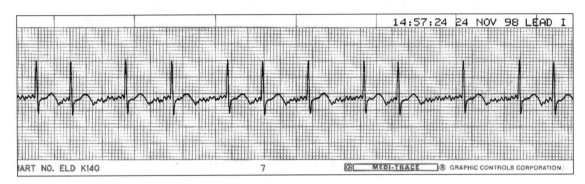

Atrial fibrillation.

○ **What is the cardiac arrhythmia?**

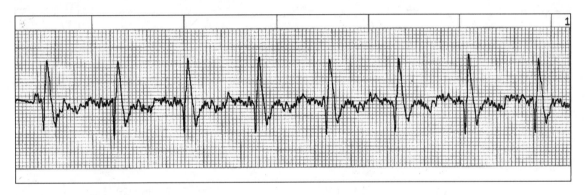

Ventricular paced rhythm with artifact.

○ **What is the cardiac arrhythmia?**

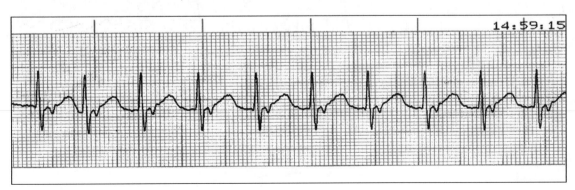

Accelerated junctional rhythm with retrograde P waves.

○   **What is the cardiac rhythm seen below?**

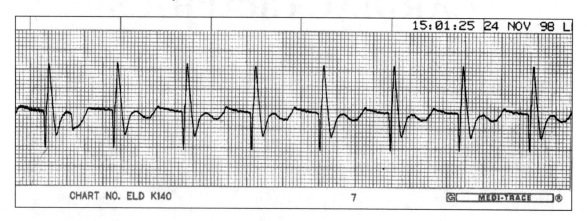

Ventricular pacemaker rhythm.

○   **What is the ECG rhythm abnormality seen below?**

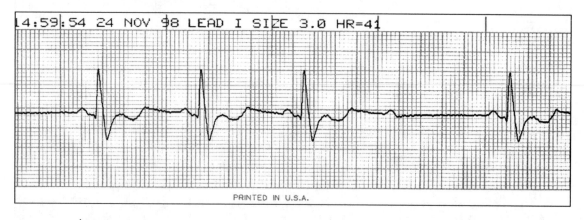

Mobitz II 2nd degree AV block.

○   **What is the ECG rhythm abnormality seen below?**

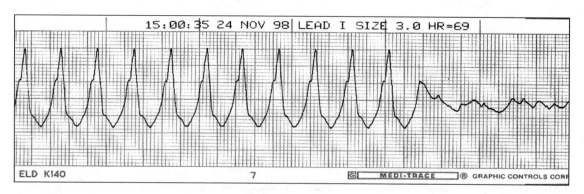

Ventricular tachycardia evolving into ventricular fibrillation.

○   **What is the cardiac arrhythmia below?**

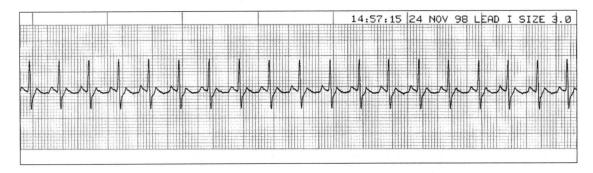

Atrial tachycardia with 2:1 conduction.

○   **What is the abnormality in the ECG seen below?**

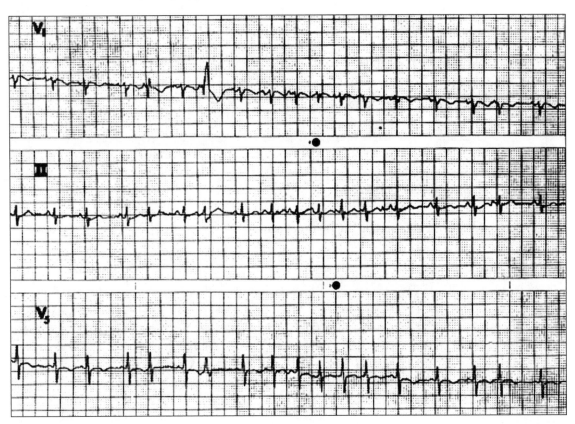

Multifocal atrial tachycardia.

○ **What is the abnormality seen in the rhythm below?**

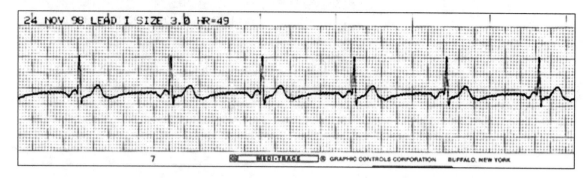

Junctional rhythm.

○ **What is the abnormality seen in the rhythm below?**

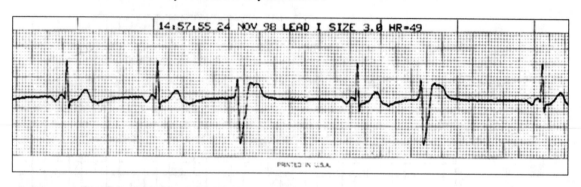

Junctional rhythm with escape ventricular beats.

○ **What is the abnormality seen in the rhythm below?**

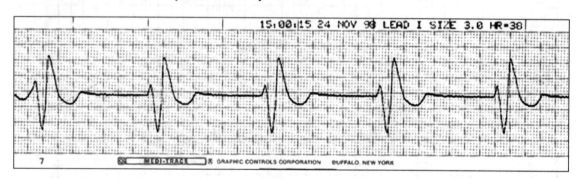

Idioventricular rhythm.

○   **What is the abnormality seen in the rhythm below?**

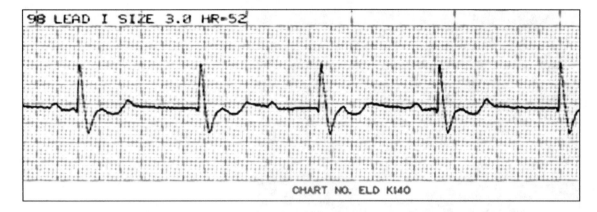

2:1 AV block.

○   **What is the abnormality seen in the rhythm below?**

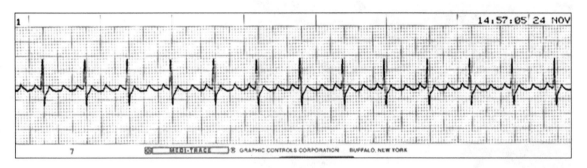

Atrial flutter.

○   **What is the abnormality seen in the rhythm below?**

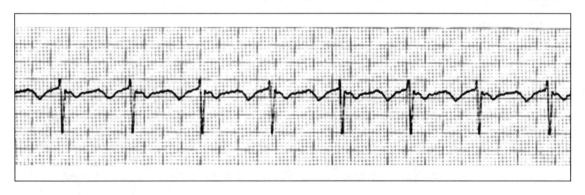

Rhythm strip erroneously mounted upside down. When viewed right-side up, it shows normal sinus rhythm.

○   **What is the abnormality seen in this two-dimensional echocardiogram?**

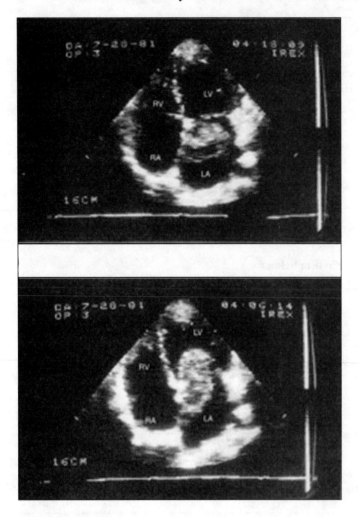

Left atrial myxoma.

○   **What is the rhythm seen below?**

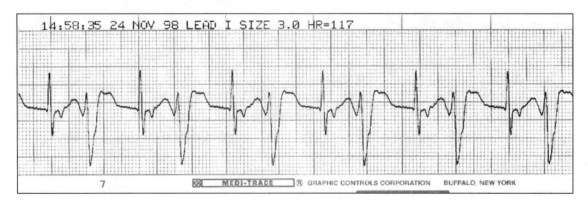

Atrial tachycardia with ventricular bigeminy.

○ **What is the rhythm abnormality seen below?**

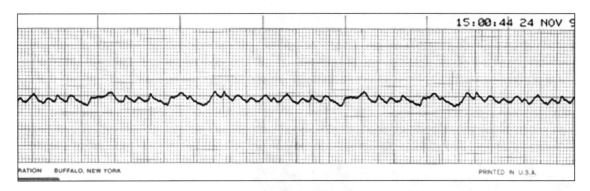

Ventricular fibrillation.

○ **What is the rhythm abnormality seen below?**

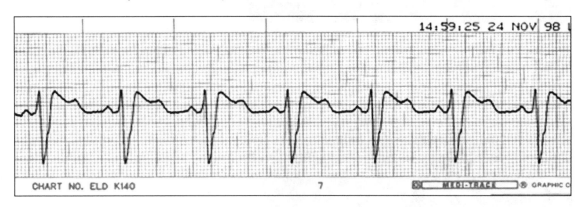

Complete heart block.

○ **What does the Doppler echocardiogram below show?**

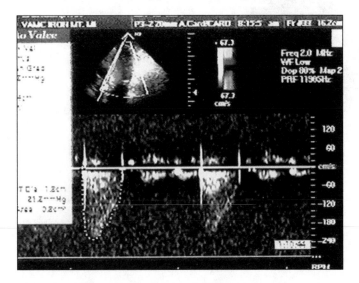

Mild aortic stenosis with a peak systolic flow velocity of 2.5 m/sec.

○   **What does the Doppler echocardiogram below show?**

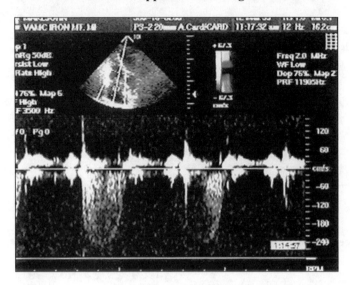

Mild tricuspid regurgitation with mild pulmonary hypertension, as evidenced by a 25 mm peak gradient across the tricuspid valve.

○   **What does the Doppler echocardiogram below show?**

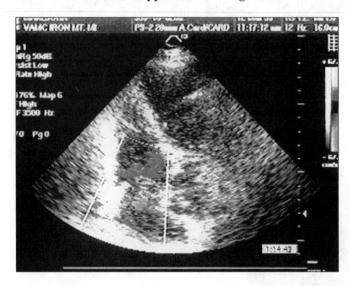

Moderate tricuspid regurgitation.

❍ **What does the Doppler echocardiogram below show?**

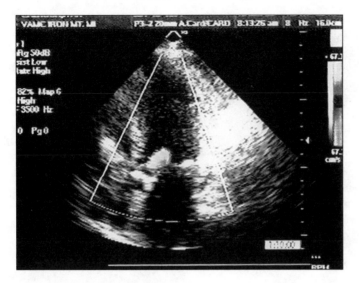

Moderate aortic regurgitation.

❍ **What does the M-mode echocardiogram below show?**

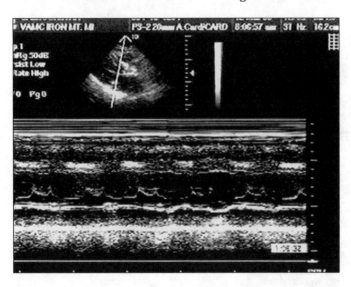

Mitral valve sclerosis with mitral annular calcification.

○   **What does the Doppler echocardiogram below show?**

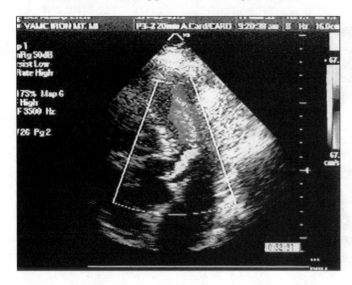

Moderate to severe aortic regurgitation.

○   **What can you say about the LV function based on the M-mode of the aortic valve shown below?**

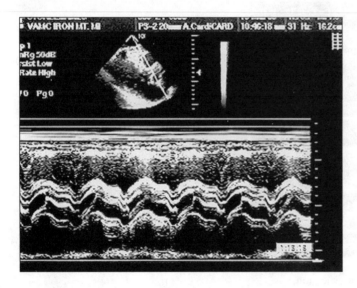

This patient has normal LV systolic function. Note the excellent aortic motion.

○ **What does this transesophageal echocardiogram of the thoracic aorta show?**

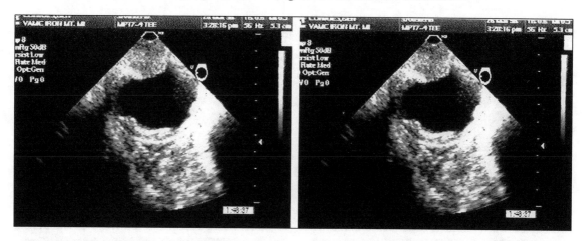

Moderate to severe aortic atherosclerosis with a large plaque in the anterior aspect of the aortic wall. Note the circumferential disease of the aorta.

○ **What does this transesophageal echocardiogram show?**

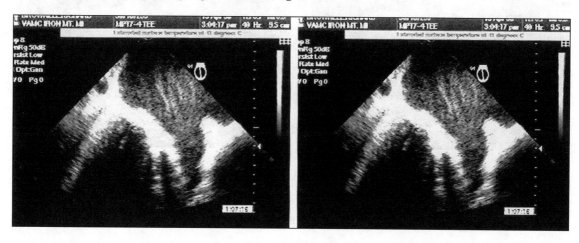

Spontaneous contrast in a large left atrium and enlarged left atrial appendage. No atrial thrombi are seen.

O   **What is seen in the transesophageal echocardiogram below?**

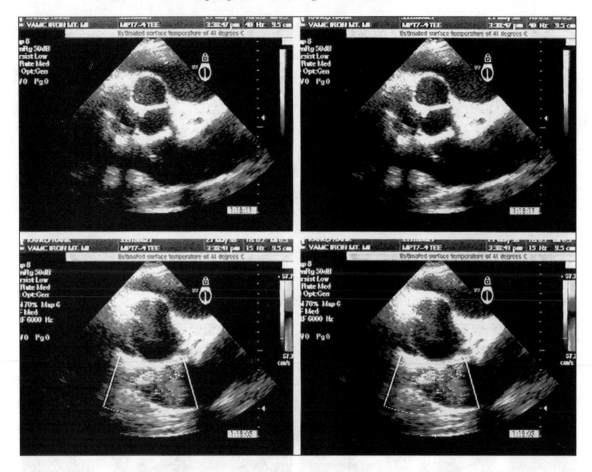

The pulmonic valve with the pulmonary artery is seen below the aorta and aortic valve. The color Doppler shows pulmonic regurgitation.

O   **What is seen in the transesophageal echocardiogram below?**

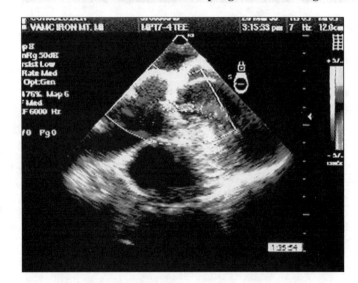

Aortic regurgitation across a very thickened aortic valve.

○   **What is seen in this transesophageal echocardiogram shown below?**

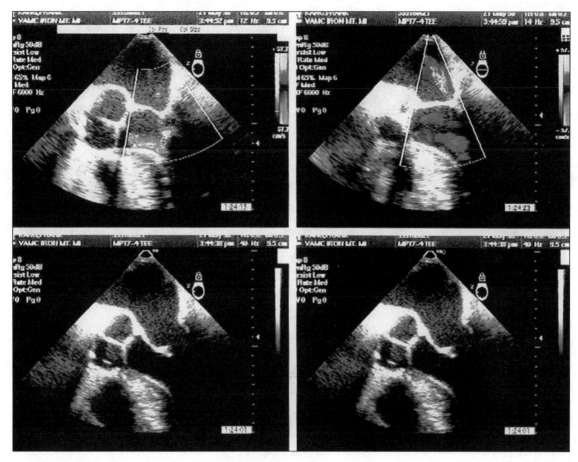

Thickened mitral valve, mild to moderate aortic regurgitation, and mild to moderate eccentric mitral regurgitation.

○   **What is seen in this Doppler echocardiogram shown below?**

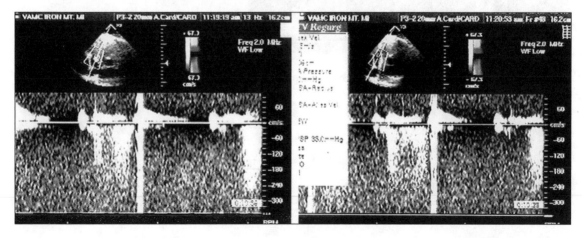

Mild to moderate tricuspid regurgitation with a peak gradient across the tricuspid valve of 36 mm Hg. This patient has mild to moderate pulmonary hypertension.

○   **What does this M-mode echocardiogram of the LV reveal about this patient's LV systolic function?**

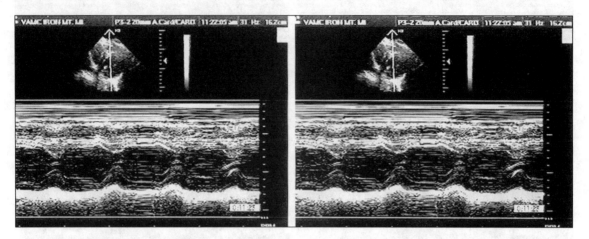

This patient's systolic function is normal.

○   **What does this M-mode echocardiogram at the aortic valve level reveal about this patient's LV systolic function?**

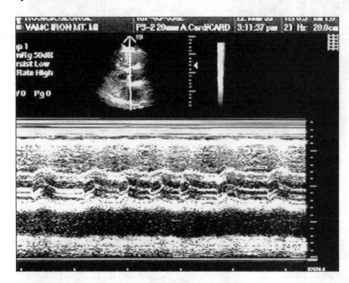

This patient's LV systolic function is poor. Note the poor motion of the aorta and the early closure of the aortic valve.

○ **What does this M-mode echocardiogram at the LV level reveal?**

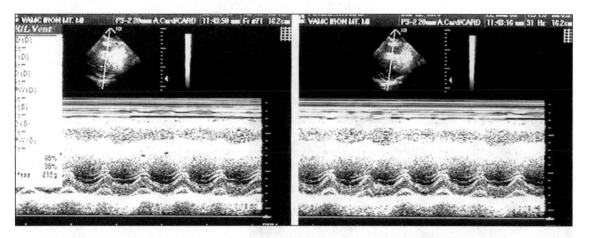

This patient has a small pericardial effusion. Note the echo-free space below the posterior wall and between the pericardium.

○ **What does this electrophysiology study show?**

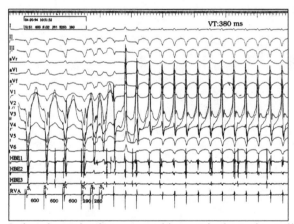

Induced sustained monomorphic ventricular tachycardia.

○ **What is the abnormality seen on this waveform tracing taken during cardiac catheterization?**

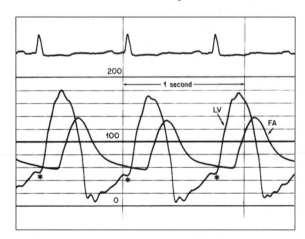

Severe aortic stenosis.

❍   **What is the abnormality seen on this Doppler echocardiogram shown below?**

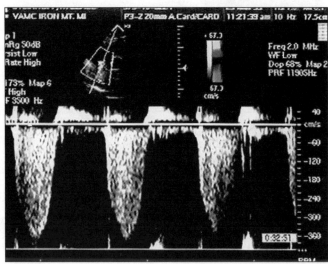

Moderate to severe tricuspid regurgitation with severe pulmonary hypertension, as evidenced by the 4 m/sec flow velocity across the tricuspid valve.

❍   **What is the interpretation of this ECG shown below?**

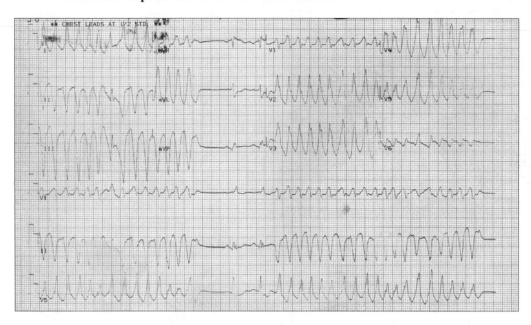

Ventricular tachycardia, most likely originating from the left ventricle.

O   **What is the interpretation of this ECG shown below?**

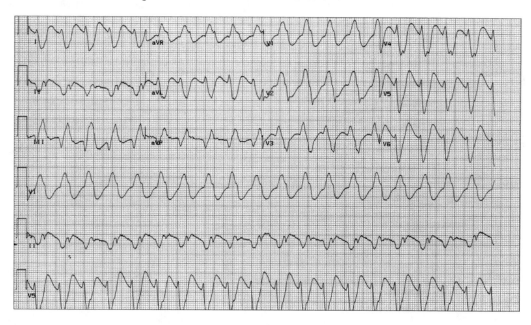

Ventricular tachycardia with hyperkalemia. Note the very wide QRS complex with the early stages of a "sine wave".

O   **What is the interpretation of the ECG shown below?**

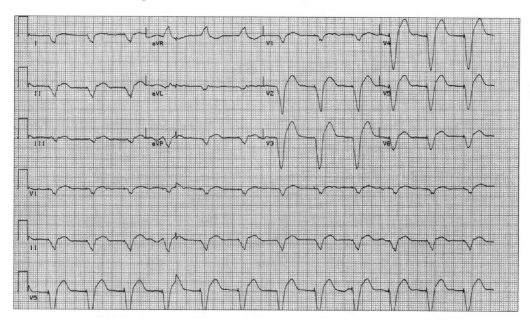

A single chamber ventricular pacemaker rhythm with 100% capture and 100% sensing. The underlying atrial rhythm is fibrillation as there are no P waves visible.

○   **What is the interpretation of the ECG shown below?**

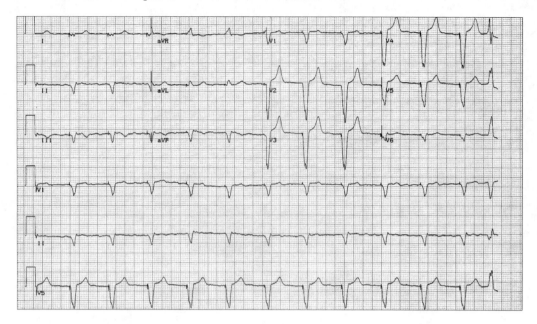

Single chamber ventricular pacemaker rhythm with 100% capture. The underlying atrial rhythm is fibrillation. This pacemaker is in VVI mode.

○   **What is the interpretation of the ECG shown below?**

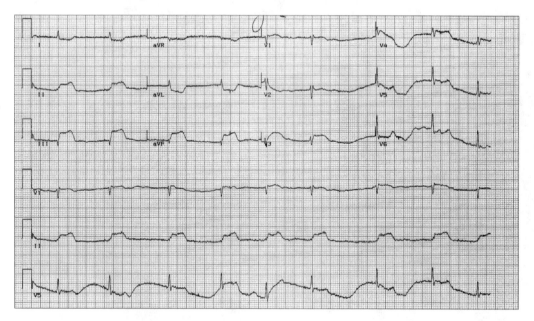

Acute inferior myocardial infarction with posterior wall involvement, atrial fibrillation with slow ventricular rate.

○   **What is the interpretation of the ECG shown below?**

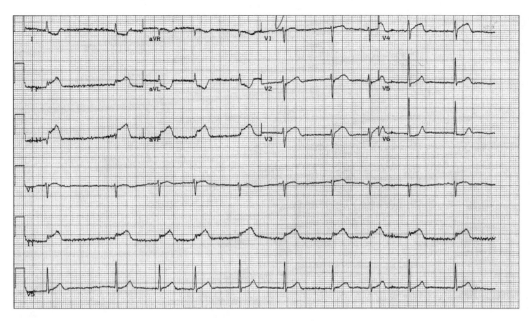

Acute inferior myocardial infarction, atrial fibrillation with slow ventricular rate.

○   **In the above ECG, does this patient absolutely have myocardial ischemia?**

Not necessarily. Patients with supraventricular tachycardia of any type with ST depression can have "ischemic" appearing ST depression without having myocardial ischemia. The ST depression can be as a result of abnormal repolarization that occurs in any tachyarrhythmia. Nonetheless, it would be incorrect to automatically assume that this patient's ST depression is not due to myocardial ischemia.

○   **What is the interpretation of the ECG shown below?**

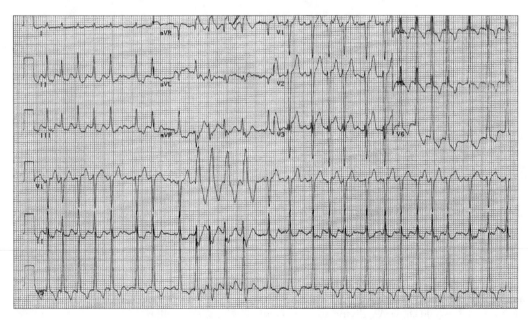

Atrial fibrillation with rapid ventricular rate of 155, LVH, and ischemic-type ST depression in the inferior and lateral leads.

O   **What is the interpretation of the ECG shown below?**

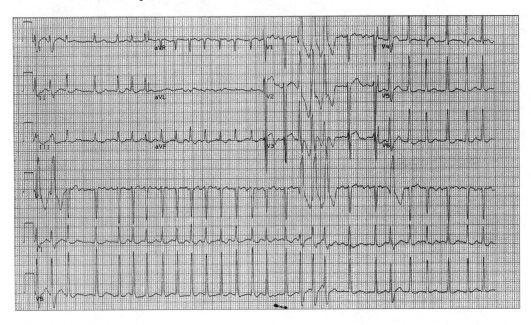

Atrial fibrillation with rapid ventricular rate, and classic example of Ashman's phenomenon. The aberrantly conducted wide-QRS complexes are not ventricular tachycardia, but aberrantly conducted impulses from the atrial fibrillation. Note the long-short-long R-R interval just preceding the Ashman's beats, a hallmark of Ashman's phenomenon.

O   **Based on the ECG shown below, does this patient have a single chamber pacemaker or a dual chamber pacemaker?**

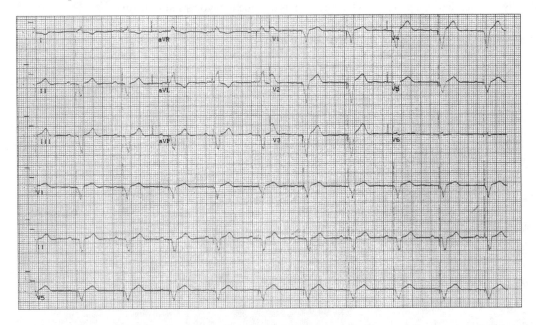

Dual chamber. Note the P waves preceding the ventricular pacer spikes and the constant P-R interval, thereby signifying a sensing of the native atrial impulses and pacing of the ventricle. A single chamber ventricular pacemaker would show AV dissociation in a patient with sinus rhythm.

O   **What is the interpretation of the ECG shown below?**

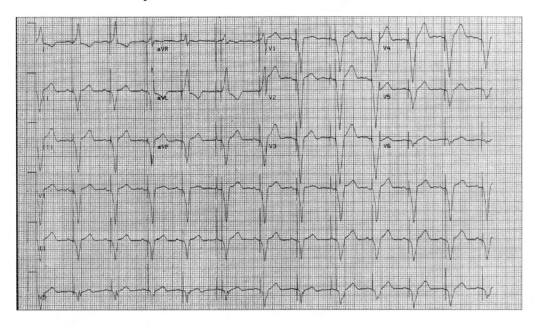

Dual chamber pacemaker in DDD mode with alternating AV sequential and AV synchronous pacing. Note the atrial sensing in the complexes without a preceding P spike prior to the P wave. The ventricle is 100% paced.

O   **What is the most likely underlying conduction abnormality in a patient with the ECG shown in the preceding question?**

Complete AV block (3rd degree).

O   **What is the interpretation of the ECG shown below?**

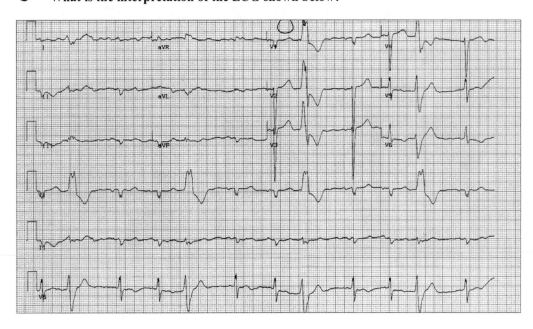

Normal sinus rhythm, left anterior fascicular block, multiple polymorphic PVC's, low voltage in the limb leads, left atrial enlargement and LVH.

○   **What is the interpretation of the ECG shown below?**

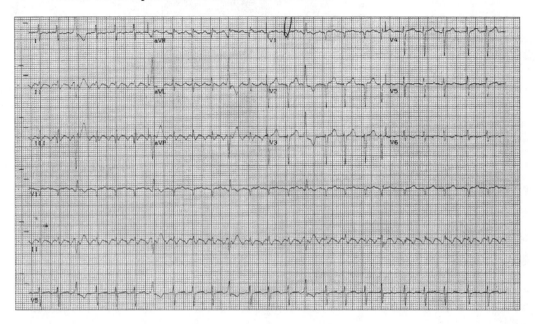

Atrial flutter with 2:1 block with aberrantly conducted complexes, old anteroseptal infarct and non-specific ST abnormality.

○   **What is the interpretation of the ECG shown below?**

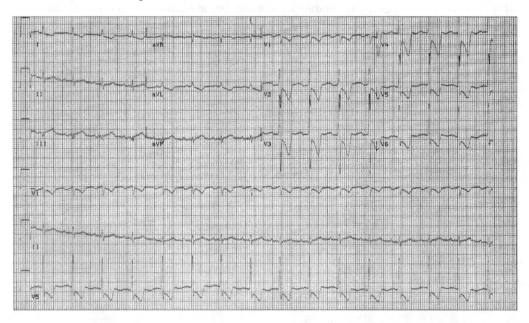

Normal sinus rhythm and profound anterolateral ST depression with T inversion, highly suggestive of a non-Q wave myocardial infarction.

○   **What is the interpretation of the ECG seen below?**

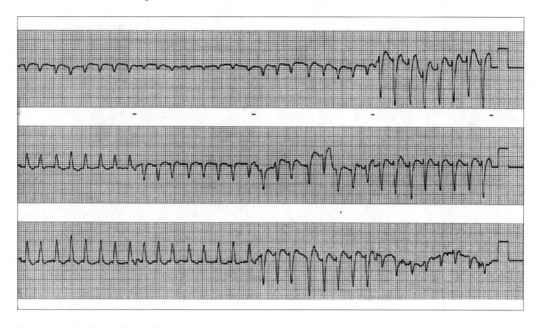

Supraventricular tachycardia.

○   **What is the interpretation of the ECG shown below?**

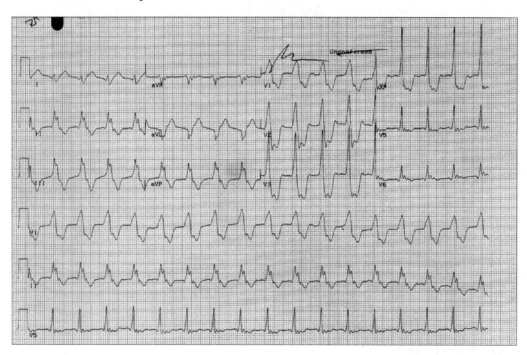

Ventricular tachycardia with a ventricular rate of 103. Note the VA conduction evidenced by the retrograde P waves, which occur in the early part of the ST segment.

○   **What is the interpretation of the ECG shown below?**

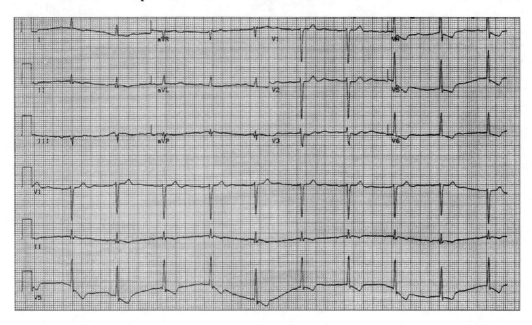

Atrial ectopic rhythm, old inferior myocardial infarction and non-specific ST-T abnormalities in the lateral leads. Note the inverted or biphasic P waves in the inferior leads.

○   **What is the interpretation of the ECG shown below?**

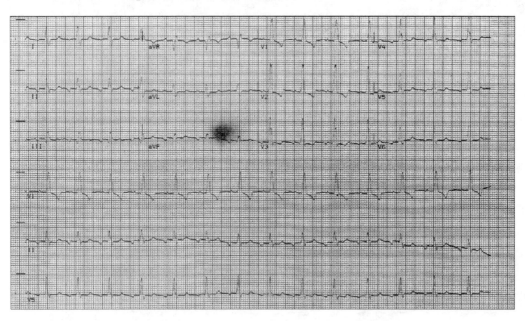

Atrial ectopic rhythm and RBBB.

○   **What is the interpretation of the ECG shown below?**

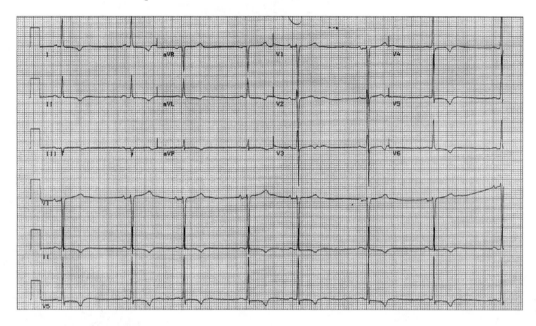

Sinus arrhythmia, a non-conducted PAC, and LVH with repolarization abnormalities. Note the P wave in the early part of the QRS of complex #5, followed by a U wave, followed by a pause.

○   **What is the interpretation of the ECG shown below?**

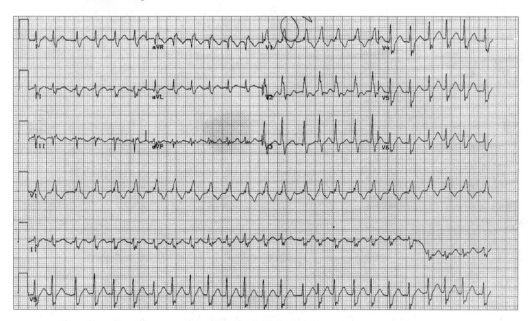

Normal sinus rhythm, RBBB and left anterior fascicular block (bifascicular block).

O   **What is the interpretation of the ECG shown below?**

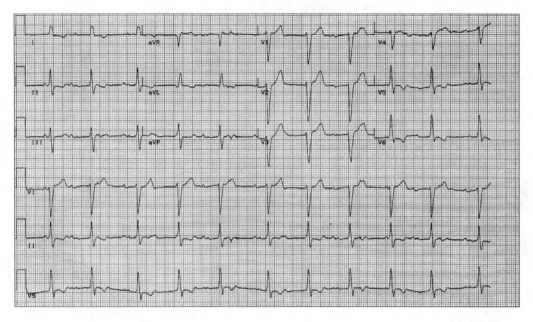

Normal sinus rhythm, 3rd degree AV block with accelerated ventricular rate.

O   **What is the interpretation of the ECG shown below?**

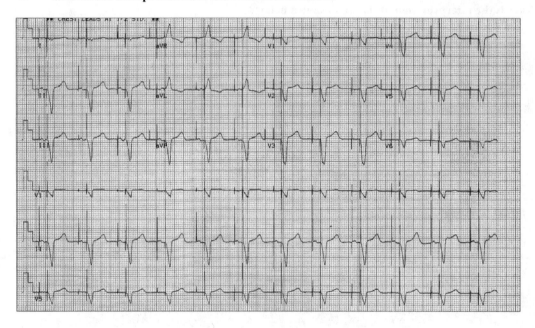

Dual chamber pacemaker rhythm with 100% pacing of both the atrium and ventricle.

○ **What is the interpretation of the ECG shown below?**

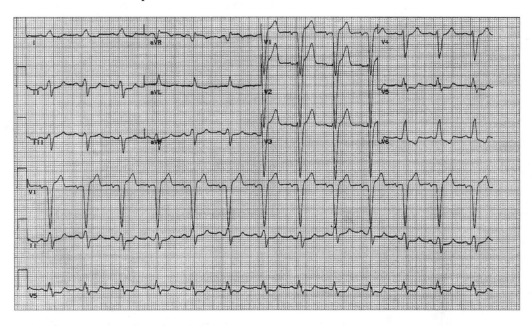

Normal sinus rhythm and LBBB with repolarization abnormalities. Note the very deep S wave in V2, measuring 33 mm, but this is 2 mm short of calling it LVH.

○ **What is the interpretation of the ECG shown below?**

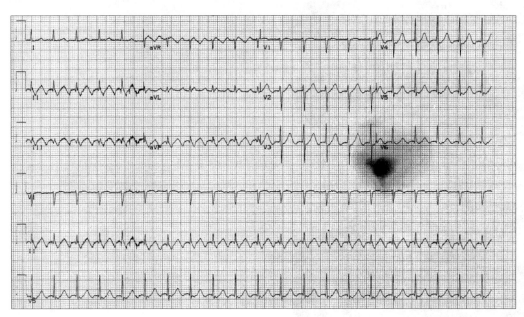

Atrial flutter with 2:1 conduction.

○ **What is the interpretation of the ECG shown below?**

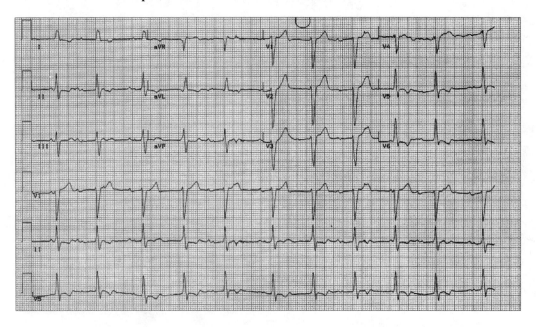

Complete heart block with left bundle branch type ventricular complexes.

○ **What is the abnormality in the M-mode echocardiogram shown below?**

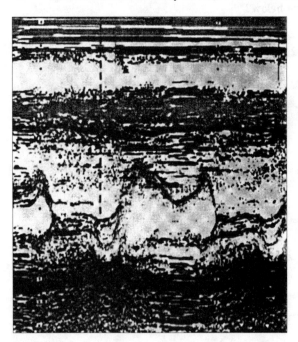

Prolapse of the posterior leaflet of the mitral valve.

○   **What is the abnormality in the echocardiogram shown below?**

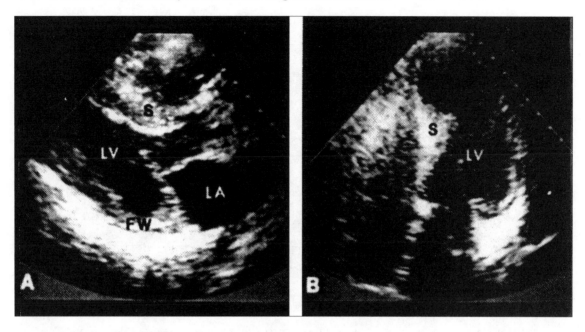

Hypertrophic cardiomyopathy. Note the very thickened septum and anterior systolic motion of the mitral valve.

○   **What is the interpretation of the ECG seen below?**

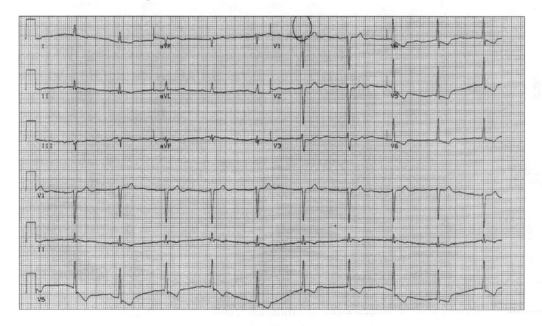

Ectopic atrial rhythm with an old inferior infarction and non-specific ST-T abnormality.

O   **What is the interpretation of the ECG seen below?**

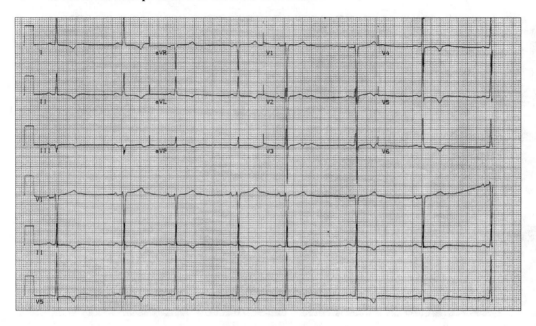

Marked sinus bradycardia with a non-conducted PAC, LVH with ST-T repolarization abnormality.

O   **What is the interpretation of the ECG seen below?**

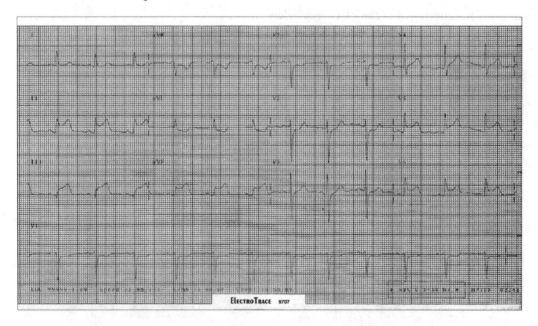

Normal sinus rhythm with an acute inferior wall myocardial infarction.

❍   **What is the interpretation of the ECG seen below?**

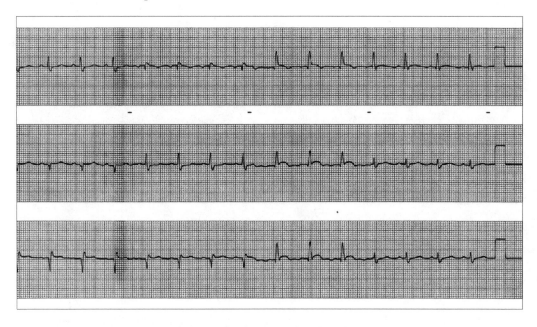

Normal sinus rhythm, RBBB, left anterior fascicular block and an acute anterior myocardial infarction.

❍   **What is the interpretation of the ECG seen below?**

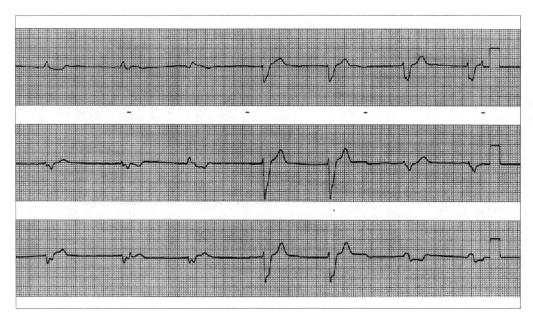

Idioventricular rhythm, rate of 40/min.

O   **What is the interpretation of the ECG seen below?**

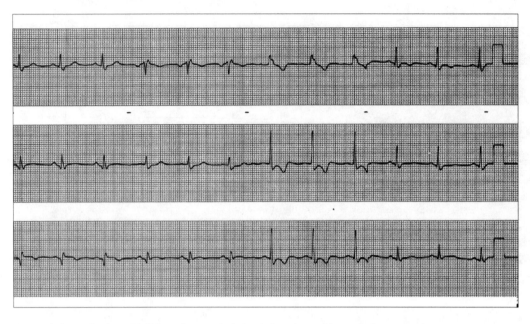

Normal sinus rhythm, RBBB and acute inferior infarction with posterior extension.

O   **What is the interpretation of the ECG seen below?**

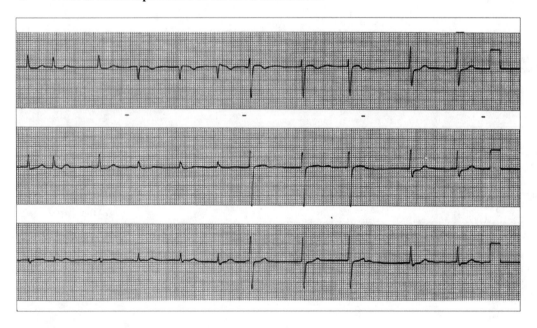

Atrial fibrillation, ventricular rate of 68/min.

BIBLIOGRAPHY

Alexander, R., Schlant, R., Fuster, V., Alexander, W., Sonnenblick, E., Hursts the Heart, Arteries and Veins, (9th Edition), McGraw Hill, 1998.

Baim, D., Grossman, W., Cardiac Catheterization, Angiography, and Intervention, (6th Edition), Lippincott, Williams & Wilkins, 2000.

Braunwald, E., Heart Disease: A Textbook of Cardiovascular Medicine, (6th Edition), W. B. Saunders Co., 2001.

Cohn, J., Management of Heart Failure, E M I S, Inc., 1990.

Falk, R., Podrid, P., Atrial Fibrillation: Mechanisms and Management, (2nd Edition), Lippincott, Williams & Wilkins, 1997.

Feigenbaum, H., Echocardiography, (5th Edition), Lea & Febiger, 1995.

Fuster, V., Ross, R., Topol, E., Atherosclerosis and Coronary Artery Disease, (2nd Edition) Lippincott, Williams & Wilkins, 2004.

Gersh, B., Rahimtoola, S., Acute Myocardial Infarction (Current Topics in Cardiology), (2nd Edition), Lippincott, Williams & Wilkins, 1997.

Kaplan, N., Lieberman, E., Clinical Hypertension, (8th Edition), Lippincott, Williams & Wilkins, 2002.

McCall, D., Rahimtoola, S., Heart Failure (Current Topics in Cardiology), Lippincott, Williams & Wilkins, 1995.

Naccarelli, G., Cardiac Arrhythmias: A Practical Approach (Clinical Cardiovascular Therapeutics Ser. Vol. 2), Futura Publishing Co., 1990.

Netter, F., Yonkman, F., Heart (The Ciba Collection of Medical Illustrations, Vol 5), Novartis Medical Education, 1978.

Patel, S., Cohn, J., Willerson, J., Handbook of Cardiovascular Clinical Trials, Churchill Livingstone, 1997.

Podrid, P., Kowey, P., Cardiac Arrhythmia: Mechanisms, Diagnosis, and Management, (2nd Edition) Lippincott, Williams & Wilkins, 2001.

Popma, J., Leon, M., Topol, E., Atlas of Interventional Cardiology, (2nd Edition) W. B. Saunders Co., 2003.

Rahimtoola, S., Valvular Heart Disease and Endocarditis (Atlas of Heart Disease, Vol. 11), Current Medicine, 1996.

Topol, E., Califf, R., Comprehensive Cardiovascular Medicine (2 Vols.), Lippincott, Williams & Wilkins, 1998.

Topol, E., Califf, R., Isner, J., Textbook of Cardiovascular Medicine, (2nd Edition) Lippincott, Williams & Wilkins, 2002.

Wagner, G., Marriott, H. J. L., Marriotts Practical Electrocardiography, (10th Edition), Lippincott, Williams & Wilkins, 2001.

Willerson, J., Cohn, J., Atlas of Ischemic Heart Disease: Clinical and Pathologic Aspects, Churchill Livingstone, 1997.

Willerson, J., Cohn, J., Cardiovascular Medicine, (2nd Edition) Churchill Livingstone, 2000.

Zipes, D., Jalife, J., Cardiac Electrophysiology: From Cell to Bedside, (4th Edition), W. B. Saunders Co., 2004.